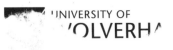

Essential Nursing Care

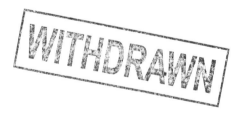

This text is dedicated to all the students from our past, present and future.

Essential Nursing Care

A Workbook for Clinical Practice

Edited by

Louise Lawson
University of Hertfordshire

And

Ian Peate
University of Hertfordshire

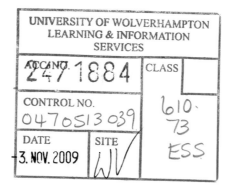
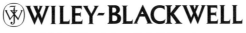
WILEY-BLACKWELL

A John Wiley & Sons, Ltd., Publication

Library of Congress Cataloging-in-Publication Data

Essential nursing care : a workbook for clinical practice / edited by Louise Lawson and Ian Peate.
    p. ; cm.
Includes bibliographical references and index.
ISBN 978-0-470-51303-3 (pbk. : alk. paper) 1. Nursing–Handbooks, manuals, etc. I. Lawson, Louise, 1960- II. Peate, Ian.
    [DNLM: 1. Nursing Care–methods–Handbooks. 2. Nursing Process–Handbooks. WY 49 E745 2009]
    RT51.E77 2009
    610.73–dc22

                                                                                           2008041817

A catalogue record for this book is available from the British Library.

Set in 10/13 Myriad MM by Aptara Inc., New Delhi, India
Printed in Singapore by Fabulous Printers Pte Ltd

1   2009

Contents

Contributor biographies

Helen Barnett RN, BSc (Hons), Pg Cert (Critical Care), PgDip (HE), FHEA

Helen Barnett graduated from the University of Hertfordshire in 1999 with a BSc (Hons) in Adult Nursing. She began her career working in cardio-respiratory medicine and coronary care. She went on to develop her interest in critical care, working in high dependency and intensive care units. She developed a particular interest in neurosciences, and worked as a Practice Development Nurse in a regional Neurosciences Critical Care Unit in East Anglia. Helen is now a Lecturer in Adult Nursing at the University of Hertfordshire and contributes to both pre- and post registration nursing programmes. She is currently in the final stages of completing her MA in Learning and Teaching. Helen continues to work as a registered nurse in her field of intensive care on a part-time basis.

Thomas Beary BSc (Hons), PGDE, Dip. HE, RN (Adult), RMN, ENB Higher Award, Advanced Diploma in the Nursing Care of Older People, FHEA

Thomas qualified as a Registered Mental Health Nurse at Claybury Hospital, Essex, in 1991 and he worked in old age psychiatry in dementia care. In 1994, Thomas worked as a senior staff nurse and junior charge nurse on an elderly acute admission psychiatry unit at the Royal Free Hospital and he was promoted to senior charge nurse in old age psychiatric rehabilitation in 1995. In 1999, Thomas undertook RN (Adult) training with Middlesex University in conjunction with the Royal Free Hospital. General nursing experiences include general and stroke rehabilitation at the Royal Free Hospital, a senior charge nurse in acute medicine at Watford General Hospital and as a discharge nurse co-ordinator with Watford and Three Rivers PCT based at West Hertfordshire Hospitals NHS Trust. Thomas is currently a Senior Lecturer in Mental Health Nursing.

Louise Lawson MA (HE), BSc Hons, RNT, RGN, EN

Louise Lawson (nee Smith) trained as an Enrolled Paediatric Nurse in 1980 in Carshalton Surrey and converted to Adult RGN in 1990 at the University College Hospital, London. Louise worked in both Saudi Arabia and Dubai as a Paediatric/Neonatal Nurse for 5 years and then returned to England to work in London and Hertfordshire specialising in Neonatal and Paediatric care. She is currently a Senior Lecturer in the School of Nursing and Midwifery and contributes to the development of clinical skills for pre-registration students and preparation for mentorship in post registration nursing. Louise is a Fellow of the Higher Education Academy.

Vijaya Rajoo Naidu RN, BSc Nursing, RNT

Vijaya has been a registered nurse for more than 20 years and has clinical experience in a wide variety of clinical and cultural settings including surgery and transplant unit, high dependency, neurosurgery, ENT and eye unit, orthopaedic, gynaecology and accident and emergency. She trained in Singapore and worked in Australia and Sultanate of Oman for a couple of years in accident and emergency department. Vijaya came to England in 1998 and worked in accident and emergency department in St Georges Hospital as an Acting Matron. She is currently a Senior Lecturer in the School of Nursing and Midwifery and predominantly contributes to post registration nursing programmes.

Ian Peate Associate Head of School, EN(G), RGN DipN (Lond) RNT, BEd (Hons), MA(Lond), LLM

Ian began his nursing a career in 1981 at Central Middlesex Hospital, becoming an Enrolled Nurse working in an intensive care unit. He later undertook 3 years student nurse training at Central Middlesex and Northwick Park Hospitals, becoming a Staff Nurse then a Charge Nurse. He has worked in nurse education since 1989. His key areas of interest are nursing practice and theory, sexual health and HIV/AIDS. He is currently Associate Head of School. His portfolio centres on recruitment and marketing and professional academic development within the School of Nursing and Midwifery.

Julie Vuolo PgDip (HE), Bsc, Dip(HE) Tissue Viability, RGN

Julie Vuolo (nee Baker) has been a registered nurse for more than 20 years and has clinical experience in a wide variety of clinical settings including medicine, surgery and elderly care. In recent years, Julie has worked in clinical practice development and nurse specialist roles and has undertaken clinical development projects with both the RCN and the King's Fund. Julie has had a special interest in skin and wound care for many years and is currently a senior lecturer in tissue viability at the University of Hertfordshire. She has written widely on tissue viability and related subjects, holds a degree in Health Care Studies and is currently studying for an MA in Learning and Teaching.

Acknowledgements

Louise Lawson

I would like to acknowledge my husband, David Lawson, and my daughters, Gabrielle and Mimi, for their loving support. In particular, I would like to express thanks to my mother, Delia, who has inspired me to write.

Ian Peate

I would like to acknowledge the help and support given to me by many people including my partner, Jussi Lahtinen, and my brother, Anthony Peate, for contributing to the artwork.

Introduction

Ian Peate and Louise Lawson

The art and science of nursing continues to grow and expand touching the lives of all directly or indirectly. This workbook aims to help and encourage you, the novice nurse, to develop important skills in key areas of care, helping you to grow into a competent practitioner and beyond. At the centre of all of this is, and quite rightly so, the patient. The National Health Service (NHS) now rejects the notion of a 'one size fits all approach' as the norm, service design and delivery is provided to patients and their families as individuals in their own home or wherever the most appropriate place for health and social care provision is to take place. Health and social care also takes place outside of the NHS, for example in the independent and voluntary care sectors where efforts are also being made to provide services that are responsive to individual needs.

The principal audience for this text are nursing students, those who are or may be thinking of undertaking NVQ/SNVQ, Access to Nursing, Cadet nursing programmes of study and those who are making a return to nursing practice, but not exclusively those mentioned. This text might be just as well suited to the shelves on a bookcase at home as it would be in a library in a university or college, or hospital ward or department. It is anticipated that the workbook will be completed alongside and in conjunction with your clinical practice and the activities discussed during your time in university or college with your teachers, mentors and peers. You might want to consider writing in the white spaces provided in the workbook; alternatively, you may wish to use your own note book. It is not anticipated that you complete the workbook in a day; it is intended to be interactive and to be completed over time.

Nurses have always been central to the provision of care, but they are making more and more of an explicit and important contribution in health and social care settings. There has been a rapid increase in technology and knowledge associated with health; nursing careers are being constantly modernised to take into account the pivotal role that nurses play in health and social care; whilst this is the case, the nurse is also working as a member of the multidisciplinary health and social care team often leading these teams but always supporting.

This workbook, produced by senior nurse educationalists from a variety of backgrounds, using a sound evidence base, begins (it can only begin) to help the novice nurse on his or her journey. Each author is dedicated to providing high quality, safe and holistic nursing care for all; underpinning this dedicated approach is the belief that each individual is a unique being, with individual distinctive needs and desires – each chapter reflects these values, attitudes and hopes.

Student nurses will become registered nurses and then go on to take up senior posts within the profession, but they have to learn their trade first, they must develop confidence, demonstrate proficiency and competence regarding a vast array of activities including high tech and high touch skills. The journey will continue even when the novice nurse becomes a registered nurse with lifelong learning being a key and required feature; it is advocated that you treat this as the first stepping stone to the successful and highly respected career – Nursing.

It is impossible for any one text to cover and address all aspects associated with the profusion of clinical skills a nurse will require to carry out nursing care in all aspects of nursing and in all venues where nursing takes place. This workbook should not be considered as an all inclusive text addressing all the skills associated with nursing, instead the reader is encouraged to identify other clinical skills they deem important that have not been addressed here and to investigate further, building up their repertoire of skills acquisition.

This text considers eight key areas of care that are interrelated and in some instances interdependent upon each other. It may be considered peculiar to include the principles of first aid in a text such as this; however, the Nursing and Midwifery Council demand that as a requirement of the common foundation programme for pre-registration nursing curricula the principles of first aid must be addressed.

The chapters

Each chapter follows a similar format, to help you with your learning. The chapters have aims associated with them, so that the reader can read with purpose; however, the text is not intended to be read from cover to cover in a prescriptive manner; indeed, it may be more advantageous to dip into an out of the chapters depending on your own needs. All chapters provide you with a list of key terms that you have to find the explanations for, in some respects this could be termed the glossary, you might have other words that you want to add to the list of key terms and this would be encouraged so, as you progress through your nursing education you can build up and develop your vocabulary as you wish.

Within the chapters are activities that have been interspaced; the activities are related to the content of the chapter and offer you the chance to note down your responses to them; in most cases there are no right or wrong answers. You are encouraged to make use of human and material resources to help you as you progress through the workbook. Case studies have been provided in an attempt to contextualise and to help you relate content to real life situations; it must be noted however, that no matter how real the content of the case study this will never beat the privilege of working with patients in their own homes or in other health and social care settings.

Some chapters provide you with a chapter quiz, placed at the end of the chapter, in an effort to reinforce and encourage learning; the answers to these tests are provided at the end of each chapter. You decide if you want to complete the quiz, the emphasis is on you and your learning; it is acknowledged that some people may not wish to complete the quiz as this is not their preferred learning style.

Chapter summaries are included and they do just that, they summarise the key and salient points that have been addressed in the chapter. Reflective practice is encouraged in all aspects of nursing and nurse education. In order to promote this important activity, every chapter provides you with a template to allow you to reflect on your practice (if you wish). The sometimes personal nature of reflection means that you can choose who you share your reflection with; you may choose not to share it with anyone, or you might want to share it with, for example, your mentor or your university or college lecturer, the choice is yours. Remember there are no right or wrong ways to reflect, what is provided in this text with regards to reflection is but one model.

Finally, each chapter concludes with a useful reading list. These comprise reference to chapters in texts, journal articles and web addresses. The websites are reliable and are from a variety of sources, for example statutory or government bodies and charitable organisations.

What's in a name?

Much debate ensued with regards to the choice of words to be used in the text, for example are you a reader or a student? Whilst it might seem pedantic to ponder over such issues, it is in fact important. Generally, you are referred to as the student; we are all students as nurses as we all have to subscribe to the concept of lifelong learning.

A more important debate developed with regards to the term patient, using any term can lead to labelling. The term patient is a common term that is often used in the NHS. There are some terms and phrases that some people might find offensive, but there maybe others who find these terms appropriate. The term patient has been chosen in the text to refer to recipients of health and social care; it is recognized that not everybody supports the use of the passive concept coupled with this term; it has the ability to accentuate the medical focus of the relationship between the person and the service being offered. By using the terms that have been employed in this text the authors are not implying that they are more suitable or accurate than any other, simply that they are commonly used by most nurses in practice.

The word 'skill' is often associated with a level of expertise in relation to an activity. The nursing profession and the public expect nurses to display a degree of proficiency and expertise in carrying out the diverse aspects of the nurse's role. This skilled performance will include proficiency in a range of motor skills, from the fundamental such as taking and recording a temperature to a more complex issue such as the passing of a urinary catheter. To function effectively in a wide range of settings, nurses must know what is expected of them and have the skills in order to link theory to practice.

This book aims to provide a context for your learning and will introduce you to the concept of clinical skills and to develop a foundation in practical nursing skills. The intention of the text is to help student's master essential nursing skills and gain an understanding of the essence of nursing practice, thereby corresponding with our philosophy which is to influence and guide learners to become responsive, proactive and professional nurses. We believe that this book will help students to realise the importance of the development of practical and clinical skills and will encourage them to dedicate more time on the acquisition of these skills. It aims to build a more explicit approach to skills development, ensuring equity and consistency of clinical learning for students working in a variety of practice settings.

We have attempted to offer you an interesting, informative and stimulating approach to the learning of some fundamental (yet complex) nursing skills; we are privileged to do this and have taken pleasure in this challenge and sincerely trust that you find the content of the chapters interesting and motivating. Most importantly, we hope that the care and support you provide to those that you have the privilege of working with will be improved as a result of your learning.

For the student companion website for this book please visit **www.wiley.com/go/lawson**

1 Principles of patient safety

IAN PEATE

> ## Aims
>
> The aim of this chapter is to introduce you to the key principles associated with patient safety and provide you with an overview of your role and function associated with this important activity.

> ## Learning objectives
>
> On completion of this chapter, you will learn to:
> - Understand what is meant by patient safety
> - Describe the pertinent issues associated with patient safety
> - Outline the factors that promote positive outcomes in respect to patient safety
> - Describe how the law impinges on issues that can affect patient safety
> - Appreciate the need for effective communication

Introduction

More than one million people are treated and cared for safely and successfully on a daily basis in the National Health Service (NHS) (National Patient Safety Agency (NPSA), 2004a). Over the years, there have been a number of technological advances and a huge increase in knowledge associated with increasingly complex healthcare systems. One outcome of the complexities associated with knowledge and technological advances is the possibility that there will be an increase in, and the likelihood that, things will and do go wrong, regardless of how dedicated, skilled and professional staff are, and unfortunately patients (and staff) do suffer harm. Patient safety encompasses a range of errors and systems failures associated with the delivery of patient care (DH, 2006a) and can include situations such as:

- Mistakes in diagnosis
- Delays in diagnosis
- Medication errors
- Treatment errors
- Problems with equipment
- Infections acquired in hospitals
- Accidents such as slips and falls

Improving patient care is a challenge for those who provide healthcare, be that in the NHS, the independent sector, the voluntary sector, in people's own homes or in hospitals. Important issues need to be taken into account when preventing things from going wrong as the result of, for example, the complex interactions between many people, the variety of skills, the use of increasingly complicated technologies and the use of numerous drugs (see Figure 1.1). The Nursing and Midwifery Council's (NMC, 2008) Code of Conduct demand that nurses and midwives work with others to protect and promote the health and well-being of those in their care, their families and carers, and the wider community; this means that people in your care should be safe. This chapter reinforces the opening tenets of the Code of Conduct. As an unqualified nurse, students of nursing are neither accountable nor answerable to the NMC. However, you have a responsibility to ensure that you make known any circumstances that you find or consider unsafe in an attempt to protect the public. These situations may concern medicine errors as well as any other unsafe or potentially unsafe practice. Chapter 2 outlines some issues associated with medicine errors.

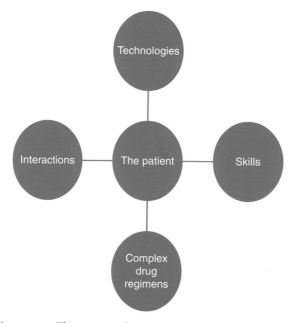

Figure 1.1 The range of complex interactions that may be associated with the administration of medicines

Activity 1.1 Key terms

Using a nursing or medical dictionary or any other resource you think may help you, begin this chapter by finding out the meaning of the key terms listed below. There may be human resources around you to help you with terms, for example, registered nurses, a pharmacist or a healthcare manager. There are blank spaces provided for you to enter your responses.

Term	Definition
Asepsis	Being free of disease producing microbes
Adverse health care event	
Bio hazardous waste	
Chain of infection	
Clinical waste	
Disinfection	
Friction	
Hazard	
Healthcare Associated Infection (HCAI)	
Healthcare Commission	
Healthcare near misses	
Infection	
Improvement notice	
Manual handling	
Microbe	

(continued)

Activity 1.1 (Continued)

Term	Definition
Microorganism	
Patient safety incident	
Pathogen	
Sharps	
Shearing	
Special measures	
Sterile	
Sterilisation	
Vaccination	
Vaccine	

When harm occurs to a patient, the effects are widespread and can be devastating from both emotional and physical perspectives to the patient, his or her family and staff. Patients may experience unnecessary pain, additional therapy or operations, and they may also have to spend additional time being cared for in the community or in a hospital. Vincent and Coulter (2002) suggest that psychological injuries such as those listed in the box below are some of the possible effects following a patient safety incident.

- Shock
- Anxiety
- Depression
- Uncertainty about recovery
- Fear of future treatments
- Disruption to work
- Disruption to family life

Source: Vincent and Coulter, 2002.

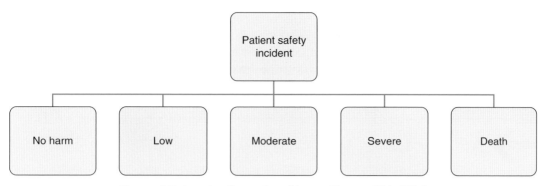

Figure 1.2 Levels of severity of harm (*Source:* DH, 2004)

Clinical staff can, as a result of the harm caused, become demoralised and in some instances disaffected. From a financial point of view, incidents that involve safety can cost the health service large amounts of money through litigation and treatment (NPSA, 2004a).

Patient safety incidents are graded according to harm. Using grading systems that are associated with the impact or harm caused to the patient can help to adopt a consistent approach to comparison and analysis of data at a national level. Figure 1.2 outlines the levels of severity related to harm and Table 1.1 provides a key to the various levels.

Table 1.1 Definitions of the levels of severity of harm (*Source:* DH, 2004c)

Level	Definition
No harm • Impact prevented	Any patient safety incident that had the potential to cause harm but was prevented, resulting in no harm
• Impact not prevented	Any patient safety incident that ran to completion but no harm occurred
Low	Any patient safety incident that required extra observation or minor treatment and caused minimal harm, to one or more patients
Moderate	Any patient safety incident that resulted in a moderate increase in treatment and which caused significant, but not permanent, harm to one or more patients
Severe	Any patient safety incident that appears to have resulted in permanent harm to one or more patients
Death	Any patient safety incident that directly resulted in the death of one or more patients

The safety of patients (and staff) concerns everyone working in clinical and non-clinical areas. A collective and systematic approach is advocated in order to have a positive impact on the quality of care and the efficiency of organisations. The NPSA has developed and produced seven steps to patient's safety; these seven steps describe the steps that are to be taken by organisations to improve safety.

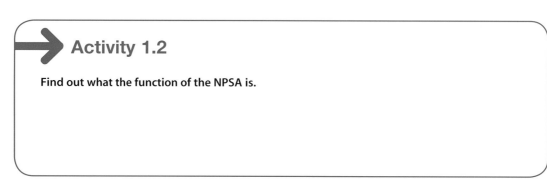

Activity 1.2

Find out what the function of the NPSA is.

The seven steps to patient safety

Using the seven steps to patient safety as a checklist can help organisations to plan activities that may help improve patient safety ensuring that care provided is as safe as possible. Table 1.2 lists the seven steps to patient safety.

Understanding what the seven steps are and what they mean can ultimately help you to help prevent harm to patients. A brief outline of each of the seven steps is provided below.

Step 1: building a safety culture

The NPSA (2004b) suggest that in order to learn about patient safety a culture of openness and fairness should be engendered. The culture should enable staff to share information freely

Table 1.2 The seven steps to safety (NPSA, 2004b)

Step	Concerned with
Step 1	Building a safety culture
Step 2	Leading and supporting staff
Step 3	Integrating risk management activity
Step 4	Promoting reporting
Step 5	Involving and communicating with patients and the public
Step 6	Learning and sharing safety lessons
Step 7	Implementing solutions to prevent harm

with the aim of improving safety levels. Staff should be encouraged to talk with colleagues and managers about incidents in which they have been involved. When incidents have been reported, investigations ought to focus upon why the incident occurred as opposed to who was involved. Staff must be supported and treated fairly when they have been involved in an incident.

Step 2: leading and supporting staff

Managers are encouraged to listen to staff and as a result you are encouraged to speak with managers and other colleagues in order to enhance safety. Try to attend any briefings or study sessions being held in the ward or department where you are working; these sessions will provide information about safety issues. Some of the issues under discussion will consider genuine safety issues that have caused concern and also issues that are known as 'near misses'.

Activity 1.3

Find out when meetings or briefings regarding safety issues are being held in the ward or department where you are working with the intention of attending one of them. Try to find out who has been appointed to act as the safety champion in your organisation; what is their role. Who in the institution where you are working is the nominated Director of Infection Prevention and Control (DIPC) and what role do they undertake? Who is the DIPC responsible to?

Step 3: integrating risk management activity

Risk management (policies, processes and procedures) must be integrated into organisational activities. It is unacceptable to manage risk at the individual level or in functional segments. Lessons learnt in one area of risk should be quickly integrated in other areas of risk.

Step 4: promoting reporting

It is important that staff are encouraged to report things that go wrong; this is a fundamental requirement for building a safer service for patients. When incidents are reported, lessons from those incidents can be learnt and improvements in patient safety made. The government has produced a report called *An Organisation with a Memory* (DH, 2000); the aim of the report was to help those working in the NHS to learn from adverse events.

The organisations where a culture of reporting is encouraged provide a safer environment for patients; this is in contrast to establishments that are swift to blame or seek retribution (DH, 2000). Staff should be congratulated when reporting incidents, not blamed or penalised if they speak out.

> ## → Activity 1.4
>
> **Go to http://www.npsa.nhs.uk/patientsafety/reporting and learn about the contents of this website. What is the aim of the National Reporting and Learning System (NRLS)? How might you go about reporting a patient safety incident? Who can report an incident?**

Step 5: involving patients and the public

Organisations that promote openness are safer organisations; patients and the public should be involved in incident investigations. Involving patients and the public in aspects associated with healthcare provision can improve patient care as well as patient safety (DH, 2000); the NHS has a duty to actively engage with the community and services users. Many patients are experts in their own condition and their expertise can be harnessed to help identify risks as well as devising ways in which to prevent further negative patient safety issues from occurring.

Being open and honest about what has happened and discussing the problem promptly in a full and compassionate manner can help patients cope better with the effects that can occur when things have gone wrong. Patients want to be involved as partners in their care and as such they should be actively encouraged to participate, for example, when making a diagnosis, making decisions concerning treatment options and discussing the risks and benefits associated with proposed treatments or therapies (Barber, 2001).

An American organisation — The Joint Commission on Accreditation of Health Organisations (JCAHO) — provides a helpful framework for engaging patients in their safety:

Speak up if you have questions or concerns and if you don't understand
Pay attention to the care you are receiving and make sure you are receiving the right treatment and medication
Educate yourself about your diagnosis
Ask for a trusted family member or friend to be your advocate
Know what medicines you are taking and why
Understand more about your health and social care organisation
Participate in all decisions around your treatment

Step 6: learning and sharing safety lessons

The focus of the government report, *An Organisation with a Memory* (DH, 2000), was to ensure that when things go wrong, when a safety incident occurs, it is not important to determine who is to blame for the incident but how and why it occurred. Analysing how often a mistake occurs, the type of mistake and level of severity of incidents and the lessons that have been learnt can help to continuously improve safety and quality of care. Understanding by sharing can assist in implementing new ways of working in order to reduce future risks.

Step 7: implementing solutions to prevent harm

When safety issues have been identified and suggestions have been made to change practice, then these suggestions must be implemented and changes made. Latest solutions and advice can be found at www.npsa.nhs.uk/advice.

Activity 1.5

Go to www.npsa.nhs.uk/advice and list some of the safer practice notices that appear on that website and think of ways in which they may be able to help you provide safer care for the people you care for.

Writing an incident report

When a patient safety issue occurs, it is usual for some form of incident report to be compiled. There are local policies and procedures (as well as the policies and procedures produced by your university or college) that must be adhered to if a complaint is raised or if there is concern about the quality, and ultimately the safety of patient care. If this is the case, then the matter must be raised immediately with the person supervising you, or to another appropriate person, for example your trade union or tutors at your university or college.

Activity 1.6

When you are next in a clinical or care area, take the time to find out what type of documentation is used to report issues that concern patient safety. Have a look at the content of the document and find out what it contains, what information is required, and what then happens to the document once it has been completed.

If you are asked to write a report or statement regarding the incident that concerns you, you must seek advice from a more senior member of staff in the clinical area or from staff at your university or college. Reports and statements must be factual; it is important to be as precise as possible, use a chronological (or sequential) approach, try to write the statement as soon as you can after the event has occurred and always ensure you keep a copy.

Practical safety concerns

The next aspects of the chapter will address issues that are often faced on a daily basis by those working in a variety of health and social care settings. In order to protect the patient and the healthcare professional, there are elements of the law that have to be adhered to, for example Health and Safety at Work Act 1974 and Control of Substances Hazardous to Health Regulations (COSHH).

Infection control

The Code of Practice for the Prevention and Control of Healthcare Associated Infections (HCAI) (DH, 2006b) arises from the Health Act 2006. The term 'healthcare associated infection' encompasses any infection by any infectious agent acquired as a consequence of a person's treatment by the NHS, or which is acquired by a healthcare worker in the course of his or her NHS duties.

For prevention and control of HCAIs to be effective, measures taken to stop and manage infection must be embedded into everyday practice; they must be applied consistently and this includes nurses, physiotherapists, doctors and other healthcare staff. All staff have a responsibility to maintain high standards of personal hygiene and to ensure that they work in a clean environment and by doing this they are helping to break the chain of infection. Wear a clean uniform everyday, wear minimal jewellery, no bracelets or wristwatches — jewellery traps microorganism and makes washing more difficult; long hair should be tied back and must be off the shoulders — loose flowing long hair has the potential to spread microorganism. Looking clean and hygienic can instil confidence in the public.

The Department of Health (2006a) states that it is important to ensure early and rapid diagnosis of an HCAI. It is also noted that all staff should demonstrate good infection control and hygiene practice; unfortunately it is not possible to prevent all infections. However, with good practice and careful hygiene it is estimated that 15–30% of HCAIs can be prevented.

The Code of Practice for the Prevention and Control of Healthcare Associated Infections (DH, 2006b) provides NHS bodies with information to enable them to plan and implement ways in which they can prevent and control HCAIs. The code outlines issues concerning ways in which organisations can ensure that patients are cared for in a clean environment where the risk of HCAI is kept low. If an NHS organisation fails to observe the code, this can result in an Improvement Notice being served to the NHS organisation by the Health Care Commission or they may be reported for significant failings and placed on 'special measures'.

Each NHS organisation must produce and adhere to policies and protocols applicable to infection prevention and control; each policy must be clearly marked with a review date. All policies must be based on the best available evidence. Specific policies associated with infection control could include, for example:

- Standard (universal) infection control precautions
- Aseptic technique

- Isolation of patients
- Safe handling and disposal of sharps
- Prevention of exposure to blood borne viruses
- Disinfection policy
- Antimicrobial prescribing

➡ Activity 1.7

Find out where the following policies are kept in the clinical or care area where you are working:

- Standard (universal) infection control precautions
- Aseptic technique
- Isolation of patients

What is the review date?

Standard (universal) infection control precautions

Standard precautions (they are sometimes called universal precautions) according to Parboteeah (2002) are implemented in an attempt to control infection. Infection control is described by Rennie-Meyer (2007) as a number of measures that are taken to prevent infections from occurring in healthcare facilities with the aim to destroy or remove sources of pathogenic microorganisms. There are several ways in which this can happen, for example:

- Interrupting the transmission of pathogens
- Protecting individuals from becoming infected

It is important to minimise, reduce and eliminate potential environmental contamination; all body fluids, including blood, must be considered potentially infectious for all patients. Effective management of blood and body fluid spillages is vital in order to prevent the transmission of infection (Peate, 2008). All staff must ensure that any spillage of blood or another body fluid is dealt with immediately. According to Rennie-Meyer (2007) and Wilson (2006) there are five key points associated with standard precautions:

1. Effective hand washing
2. Personal effective equipment
3. Safe handling and disposal of sharp instruments
4. Safe disposal of waste (including linen)
5. Decontamination of equipment

Standard precautions represent the standard of care that should be used routinely with every patient in an effort to minimise the spread of pathogens between patients and staff and also between staff and patients; these are infection control precautions.

Waste disposal

Clinical waste may be contaminated with body fluids and blood and because of this there will be microorganisms present. Clinical waste must be separated from non-clinical waste and disposed of safely in accordance with policy and protocol to prevent harm to other patients, staff or visitors.

Sharps must also be disposed of safely and small sharps bins are available that can allow you to dispose of used sharps immediately, for example when at the patient's bedside. The safe disposal of sharps is the responsibility of the user (Harriss and Cook, 2008). Never resheath a needle or over fill a sharps bin; to do so increases the risk of harm.

Activity 1.8

Check the policy and procedure in your place of work that is related to the safe disposal of clinical waste. What does it say about the colour of bags to be used for certain categories of waste? Is there only one type of sharps bin in the care area; what other types are there; what are they to be used for?

Personal protective equipment

The correct use of personal protective equipment (PPE) is another way of preventing HCAIs. PPE includes gloves, aprons and face protection and the use of this equipment will, if used correctly and appropriately, protect you and your uniform from exposure to microorganisms during procedures or episodes of care provision. The equipment forms a barrier between you and, for example, the patient's bodily fluids. PPE will become contaminated and it is vital that it is removed as soon as possible after the activity has been completed. The law states that each employer must provide PPE for all staff, and it is also important that you use it correctly; you have a duty to do this.

> ### ➡ Activity 1.9
>
> **What PPE is available where you work; do you know how to access it and do you know how to use it?**

Hand hygiene

Pittet *et al.* (2000) suggest that hand hygiene is one of the most effective measures likely to reduce HCAI. This most essential component of effective infection programmes, hand hygiene, means that those who engage in it must ensure that they use the correct technique in an attempt to ensure that all surfaces of the hands receive contact with the decontaminating agent, for example with the use of soap and water or alcohol gel (Gould and Drey, 2008).

The hands of clinical staff are the most common vehicle of spreading microorganisms between patients. Hands may become contaminated during everyday routine procedures as well as those procedures that may be in contact with blood and bodily fluids. It is vital therefore that staff know when to decontaminate hands so that the transfer of microorganisms is reduced or prevented.

There are two methods that can be used to decontaminate the hands — liquid soap and water or disinfectant hand rub. Liquid soap and water remove dirt and organic matter, as well as microorganisms you may have acquired on your hands; these are known as transient flora. Disinfectant hand rubs offer an alternative to liquid soap and water. They are an easy and effective way of decontaminating your hands, but your hands must not be contaminated with organic matter. Hand rubs can be used at the patient's bedside. When working in the community, they play an important part in hand hygiene.

> ### ➡ Activity 1.10
>
> **Where in your place of work are disinfectant hand rubs available? What do hand hygiene posters in your care area say — what message are they trying to get across?**

It is important that if you have any cuts or scratches they are covered by a waterproof plaster; do not leave any cuts or scratches uncovered. A consequence of washing your hands often is that they may become dry; if this is the case use a moisturiser — you should avoid using shared pots of moisturiser. Nails should be kept clean and short: long nails or false nails can trap microorganisms; nail polish and false nails are not allowed.

When to wash hands

Hands must be cleaned properly as microorganisms can be picked up at any time putting patients at risk. Hands should be cleaned before:

- Starting work
- You touch the patient's equipment or furniture

- Touching patients or their belongings
- Handling food or drinks

It is just as important to ensure that you clean your hands to avoid spreading microorganisms after:

- Handling dirty linen
- Handling waste
- Touching a patient or his or her belongings
- Removing gloves
- You touch patient equipment or furniture

There are also other instances when the hands must be cleaned properly and these are after:

- Finishing your shift
- Blowing your nose
- Using the toilet
- Touching anything dirty
- Coughing or sneezing into your hands

How to clean hands

Often the correct way for cleaning hands is taken for granted and it is assumed that as adults we know how to clean our hands properly. Whilst hands may not always look dirty they may in fact be harbouring a range of microorganisms; this may be particularly the case if they have been in contact with anything that is contaminated, for example after handling waste. This aspect of the chapter describes the correct technique for cleaning hands using soap and water and alcohol hand rub.

Figure 1.3 provides diagrammatic representation associated with soap and water hand washing and alcohol rub hand hygiene for visibly clean hands.

Activity 1.11

With your colleagues' permission watch them clean their hands using either soap and water or disinfectant hand rub, and observe their technique during the procedure. As the process progresses, note if they have completed each of the steps below. If a step is not done properly, take notes on what you have seen. Then ask your colleagues to watch you and do the same activity. Discuss what you all have observed and compare notes.

Step	Completed?	Notes/observation
Palms and backs of hands	Yes/No	
Between fingers	Yes/No	
Nails	Yes/No	
Thumbs	Yes/No	
Fingertips	Yes/No	
Wrists	Yes/No	

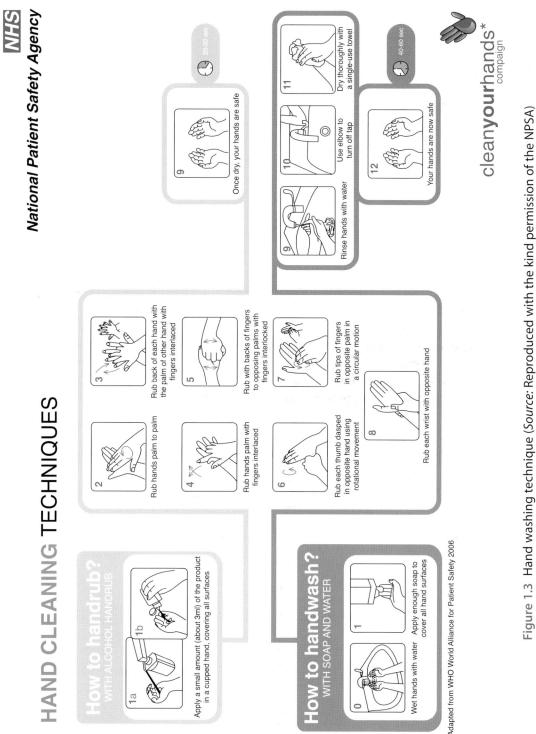

Figure 1.3 Hand washing technique (*Source*: Reproduced with the kind permission of the NPSA)

Gould *et al.* (2007) have noted that despite the fact that alcohol hand rubs are being widely promoted to increase the frequency of hand hygiene in the UK, this does not appear to have been accompanied by convincing decreases in rates of HCAI. Further research is needed with respect to this method of hand decontamination.

Aseptic technique

All clinical procedures should be performed in a manner that maintains and promotes the principles of asepsis. All people who undertake procedures that require aseptic technique should be provided with education, training and assessment in relation to the activity. The following are guidelines to be used in using aseptic technique to dress a wound. The procedure can be used in a hospital or community setting with minor modifications; for example, in a hospital setting a dressing trolley will be available and this may not be the case in a person's own home. The procedure may need to be adjusted to ensure that it complies with local policy and procedure:

- Explain the proposed procedure to the patient.
- Ideally, use a treatment room to perform the dressing change; if this is not possible ensure that the environment surrounding the bed is appropriately prepared.
- Wash hands using correct technique.
- The dressing trolley should be washed and dried according to policy; disinfection according to policy should also be undertaken.
- Equipment should be collected and prepared on the bottom shelf of the trolley; the equipment should be sterile and, if appropriate, expiry dates on all materials should be checked to ensure that they are in date and also to make certain that they are intact with no leakage.
- During the procedure the patient should be observed for signs of distress and anxiety and action taken to alleviate anxiety; for example, explain what is happening and what is to happen.
- Ensure that the bed is adjusted to a suitable level so as to reduce any risk of back injury and to promote comfort.
- Position the patient in such a way that they are comfortable and also so that you are able to access the wound to be dressed.
- The patient's clothing should be adjusted so that the wound is exposed enough to be dressed safely; at all times the patient's dignity must be protected.
- The patient must be given an explanation of what is happening and what is to happen.
- A plastic apron should be worn to prevent cross infection from uniform to wound.
- Wash hands using correct technique.
- The outer package of the dressing pack should be opened and the contents slipped out on to the top of the shelf of the trolley; this will then act as the sterile field.
- The patient's outer dressing is loosened.
- Wash hands using correct technique; at this stage it may be appropriate to use alcohol hand rub.
- The sterile field is opened out — touching it as little as possible; other equipment to be used is also slipped out of their packs on to the surface; saline (if this is to be used) is poured out into the gallipot that has come as a part of the dressing pack.
- Hands are decontaminated using the alcohol hand rub.
- Remove the wound dressing using the disposable bag in such a way that the hands do not touch the wound or its dressing.

- Attach the used bag to the side of the trolley.
- At this stage sterile gloves may be applied depending on policy.
- The wound is then cleaned and dressed according to the care plan; assessment is made of the wound and evidence of wound healing to be noted.
- A dressing is applied and secured in such a manner that will provide an environment that will promote optimum wound healing.
- The patient is made comfortable and any patient education required is given.
- All used equipment is disposed of in accordance with policy and procedure.

The procedure, findings and any other information must be documented in the patient's care plan and if appropriate a verbal report to the person in charge may be needed.

To reiterate, the guidelines provided here are just that, guidelines. Local policy and procedure must be adhered to in order to provide safe and effective care. The aim is to prevent infection and to promote wound healing. It is important to have an understanding of the physiology of wound healing as well as the factors that can influence this. Furthermore, an appreciation of wound assessment, choice of wound dressings and local policy is vital if care is to be effective and above all safe. Chapter 7 discusses the principles of skin care and includes issues associated with wound healing.

Levels of decontamination

There are three levels of decontamination:

- Cleaning
- Disinfection
- Sterilisation

Cleaning

Cleaning is the removal of dirt, dust and other organic matter using water and detergent. Approximately 80% of microorganisms will be removed if the item being cleaned is dried, but it must be dried thoroughly. This method is suited to any item that comes into contact with intact skin, for example beds, chairs, non-invasive monitoring equipment and intravenous pumps. If an item is to be cleaned that has been contaminated with body fluids or excretia, for example a commode, then a disinfectant solution such as hypochlorite is needed. Cleaning is the first step to decontamination by disinfection or sterilisation.

Disinfection

Disinfection removes microorganisms to a level at which they are no longer harmful; it does not, however, have any effect on spores. There are two methods of disinfection:

- Heat, i.e. the bedpan washer
- Chemical, i.e. chemicals used to disinfect instruments such as an endoscope

For disinfection to be effective, the items to be disinfected must be cleaned first.

Sterilisation

This method of decontamination is effective in destroying all microorganisms including spores. The preferred method of sterilisation is by autoclave. Just like disinfection, for this method to be effective all items must be thoroughly cleaned first.

Manual handling

Manual handling is defined by the Health and Safety Executive (HSE) (2002) as the act of transporting or supporting of a load (including the lifting, putting down, pushing, pulling, carrying or moving thereof) by hand or bodily force. A load is any object or person that must be moved; the load does not necessarily have to be heavy. Some examples of activities that constitute manual handling can be found in the box below.

- Lowering a load
- Rocking a load
- Pulling a load
- Lifting a load
- Pushing a load
- Supporting a load
- Rolling a load

Many activities carried out on a daily basis involve manual handling, at home and in the work place, for example lifting boxes, carrying children, turning a mattress. In health and social care settings this is also true; therefore, it is important to understand how to undertake manual handling safely and effectively in order to prevent injury.

There are some areas of the body that are prone to injury more than others:

- The upper limbs — including the arm, hand, wrist, thumb and finger.
- The torso — including the lower back.
- The lower limbs.

Activity 1.12

The results of a back injury can impact on various aspects of an individual's life. See if you can describe what impact may occur on the five aspects of life outlined in this table as a result of a back injury.

Aspect of life	Impact
Financial	
Social	
Domestic	
Professional	
Family life	

The back is the most likely part of the body to be injured in a manual handling incident. The spine (made up of 24 vertebrae) needs to support the head, upper parts of the body, the pelvis and the legs; this important supporting structure needs to be flexible, strong and stable. Back injuries occur when flexibility, strength and stability are compromised.

Risk management — manual handling

It is important to manage and assess risk when completing manual handling tasks. In almost every activity of living, we engage in risk taking and we usually make choices about the risks we take. We usually weigh up factors that enable us to make decisions; the outcome of the weighing up of the factors means that we either take the risk or we do not.

Risk assessment is the process of considering the potential dangers that may be associated with the activity to be undertaken. In order to understand this, there are three terms associated with risk that need to be defined:

1. Hazard — a situation or activity that might lead to harm.
2. Harm — the damage or injury caused by the hazard.
3. Risk — the likelihood and severity of the potential harm (high or low).

There are processes available to help when assessing risk and these are steeped in law. Two key aspects of legislation — the Manual Handling Operation Regulations 1992 and the Management of Health and Safety at Work Regulations 1999 — are the most relevant. The regulations set out the responsibilities for both employers and employees in avoiding unnecessary risks when manual handling. There is a three-stage framework associated with manual handling tasks that employees are obliged to apply:

1. Avoid — avoid hazardous manual handling tasks; can the activity be carried out in another way?
2. Assess — assess activities that can be avoided; what are the dangers associated with the task?
3. Reduce — reduce the risk of injury from the task to be carried out; how can the identified dangers be reduced?

In assessing a manual handling task, the following five headings, TILEO, can help you to consider all the aspects of the situation in detail:

Task
Individual
Load to be moved
Environment
Other factors in this case to be considered

The TILEO framework can be of value in identifying the dangers in manual handling tasks and to help explore ways to reduce risks. The TILEO framework can be applied to everyday activities at work or whilst going about daily activities.

> ## ➜ Activity 1.13
>
> **See if you can find evidence of the TILEO framework at use in your work place.**

Remember, you should always avoid performing a hazardous task. Always assess the situation and try to reduce the risk by finding a safer way of doing it.

Safer handling principles

It is important to note that there is no single correct way to undertake any manual handling activity; an ergonomic approach considers manual handling as a whole taking into account a range of relevant factors — the task, the environment and individual capability. Ergonomics according to Parboteeah (2002) is the study of the relationship between the working environment and the people within it. There are many factors that will impinge on the task to be carried out; for example, physical differences will affect individual risk factors, which in turn will affect the way we need to move. Table 1.3 provides tips and suggestions associated with two manual handling activities.

Patient handling

This aspect of the chapter can only provide some insight into the complex issues associated with manual handling of patients in health and social care settings. The reader is strongly advised to seek further understanding from a range of human and material resources to ensure that activities are safe. The aim should be to avoid all manual lifting in all but exceptional or life-threatening circumstances.

Each patient must be individually assessed. Assessment must be undertaken by a competent practitioner who must take into account individual needs, capabilities and circumstances. Alongside this, the person undertaking the assessment must pay due regard to staff, carers and patient safety. Assessment and any decisions to be taken should involve the patient if possible.

When assessment has been undertaken, a problem-solving approach should be implemented; this will include the consideration of a variety of handling methods and equipment to reduce the risk of injury. At all times patient independence should be encouraged. A written plan following assessment should be produced which must be reviewed at regular intervals or when the patient's condition dictates. No member of staff should be expected to put his or her own safety at risk by lifting manually. Hoists, sliding aids and other specialist equipment should be used after a thorough assessment has been undertaken. Individual risk assessment must follow safer handling principles.

Employees must take reasonable care of their own health and also be aware that they have a responsibility to care for the health of others whose safety may be affected by their actions or omissions when they are involved in manual handling operations; they must also attend any training that is related to moving and handling activities (Harriss and Cook, 2008). Staff must observe safe systems of work and use safety equipment, promptly reporting any defects in handling and equipment aids; any unsafe equipment must be taken out of service and labelled as such. Prior to using equipment such as a hoist or other lifting aid, the user should be familiar with the manufacturer's instructions for use and they must comply with these instructions (Pittet et al., 2000). It is also a requirement of staff to ensure that they wear suitable clothing and footwear to undertake manual handling safely: flat supportive footwear with a non-slip sole is required; trousers or culottes should be worn as opposed to skirts or dresses; tops or tunics should be non-restrictive and allow ease of movement.

Table 1.3 Tips and suggestions associated with two manual handling activities

Activity to be undertaken	Tips and suggestions
Lifting a load from the floor	Lifting a load from the floor is one of the more difficult sorts of manual handling task you may carry out. If possible, avoid carrying out the task manually, use machinery or approach the task in a different way. If it cannot be avoided, these steps may be helpful. ● **Adopt a stable base** — place the feet on either side of the load with one foot slightly in front of the other and point in the direction you want to go ● **Adopt a posture appropriate to the task** — maintain the natural 'S' curve of the spine as you bend your knees. Lean slightly forward to take hold of the load. If you start to feel uncomfortable stop and reassess the task ● **Get a firm grip** — grip the load firmly and try to keep the arms within the base created by your feet ● **Come up smoothly** — ensure a stable base throughout the lift, keep the load close to you, push up through your leg muscles, brace the stomach muscles and breath out gently, raise the chin slightly as you begin to come up ● **After the lift** — do not twist or stoop, beware of the arch in your back ● **Lowering the load to the floor** — in essence the issues are the same but in reverse
Team handling	Lifting or carrying a load with others may cause problems. When two or more people lift or carry a load between them, there are some additional risks. Always say 'ready, steady, lift' when lifting — this is safer as everyone lifts at the same time. ● **Is the load too heavy?** ● **Beware of height differences; this can affect how much of the load any one individual has to manage** ● **Can everyone see where they are going?** ● **Can everyone get a good grip on the load? Some parts of a load maybe harder to grip than others** ● **Does everyone start to lift at the same time?**

→ Activity 1.14 Reflection

Take some time when in clinical practice to reflect on the issue of patient safety; choose an activity that you can use to reflect upon. In the box below write what happened, how you felt, and what you would do differently (if anything) next time you are involved in the promotion of patient safety:

What happened?

How did it make you feel?

What would you do differently (if anything) next time?

Case Studies: Consider the case study below and discuss some of the issues with your mentor or supervisor at work.

Case study 1.1

Mary Jones, a 67-year-old, was being cared for in the community. Mrs Jones was a terminally ill patient who had breast cancer. She was due for a visit from the community nursing services one evening to assess her pain, but the visit (due to a variety of factors) did not occur. This resulted in Mrs Jones being in unnecessary pain until the next day when the visiting nurse noticed the visit had not occurred and her pain control medication was altered to control her pain.

The patient safety issues identified in this case study could be graded as low on the severity of harm grading scale.

Chapter summary

This chapter has introduced, and only introduced, some important issues that will impinge on both patient and staff safety. If the issues discussed are applied in the appropriate ways then this can help to prevent harm and injury to yourself and those you care for. By understanding the contents of this chapter, you can use your skills and insight to enhance the provision of care. It is not possible in a chapter of this size to address all issues concerning patient safety, and the reader is advised to read other texts and consult further in an attempt to build upon what has been provided here.

It is important that if at any stage you are in doubt about any element of patient safety (no matter how trivial you think it is) you must seek advice and support from others. Never put your patient, and indeed never put yourself, at risk of harm or injury.

Answers to Activities

Activity 1.1 Key terms

Using a nursing or medical dictionary or any other resource you think may help you, begin this chapter by finding out the meaning of the key terms listed below. There may be human resources around you to help you with terms, for example, registered nurses, a pharmacist or a health care manager. There are blank spaces provided for you to enter your responses.

Term	Definition
Asepsis	Being free of disease producing microbes
Adverse health care event	An event or omission arising during clinical care and causing physical or psychological injury to a patient (this phrase is being replaced by the phrase patient safety incident)
Bio hazardous waste	Items that are contaminated with body fluids, i.e. blood, excrement, body fluids, secretions
Chain of infection	The sequence of events that results in the passing of infection from one person to another
Clinical waste	Waste that is clinical waste as defined by the Controlled Waste Regulations
Disinfection	The process of becoming clean
Friction	The rubbing of one surface against another
Hazard	Anything that can cause harm
Healthcare Associated Infection (HCAI)	A HCAI is an infection that develops as a direct result of any healthcare treatment. The infection is not present when a patient begins the healthcare treatment
Healthcare Commission	An independent organisation that exists in England and Wales to promote improvements in the quality of healthcare and public health in England and Wales
Healthcare near misses	A situation in which an event or omission, or a sequence of events or omissions, arising during clinical care fails to develop further, whether or not as the result of compensating action, thus preventing injury to a patient
Infection	A disease state that is caused by the invasion and growth of microbes in and on the body
Improvement notice	A legal power handed to the Healthcare Commission placing compulsory duties on trusts to improve performance
Manual handling	The act of transporting or supporting of a load (including the lifting, putting down, pushing, pulling, carrying or moving thereof) by hand or bodily force.

Activity 1.1 (*Continued*)

Term	Definition
Microbe	A microorganism
Microorganism	A small living plant or organism that can only be seen by a microscope
Patient safety incident	Any unintended or unexpected incident that could have or did lead to harm for one or more persons receiving care (this phrase will replace the following phrases — adverse event, adverse incident, clinical incident, medical error, clinical error, medical mistake)
Pathogen	A microbe that is harmful and can cause infection
Sharps	Sharps are items that could cause cuts or puncture wounds. They include needles, hypodermic needles, scalpels and other blades, knives, infusion sets, saws, broken glass, and nails.
Shearing	When skin sticks to a surface and the muscle slides in the opposite direction that the body is moving
Special measures	An urgent means of acting to protect patients
Sterile	The absence of all microbes
Sterilisation	The process of destroying all microbes
Vaccination	Giving a vaccine to a person in order to produce immunity to an infectious disease
Vaccine	A preparation that contains dead or weakened microbes

Activity 1.2

Find out what the function of the NPSA is.

You may have discovered that the NPSA established in 2001 was created by the government to coordinate the efforts of all those involved in healthcare, and more importantly to learn from patient safety incidents that have occurred in the NHS. Other providers of healthcare, for example the independent sector have their own arrangements in place to ensure safety of patients.

Activity 1.3

Find out when meetings or briefings regarding safety issues are being held in the ward or department where you are working with the intention of attending one of them. Try to find out who has been appointed to act as the safety champion in your organisation; what is their role. Who in the institution where you are working is the nominated Director of Infection Prevention and Control (DIPC) and what role do they undertake? Who is the DIPC responsible to?

Meetings/briefings — frequency and content will vary depending on individual trusts.
Safety champions undergo a specified amount of training to carry out their role effectively; they primarily act as role models, promoting the prevention and control of infection within their team and their department or ward.
The role of the DIPC is multifaceted and includes:

- Being a member of senior management — (producing Board and Chief Executive reports)
- Possessing professional credibility (having special expertise)
- To act as a reporting line for the infection control team
- To implement policy
- To performance manage
- To allocate resources

The DIPC is responsible to the infection control team within the organisation

Activity 1.4

Go to http://www.npsa.nhs.uk/patientsafety/reporting and learn about the contents of this website. What is the aim of the National Reporting and Learning System (NRLS)? How might you go about reporting a patient safety incident? Who can report an incident?

The aim of the NRLS is to promote comprehensive national learning about patient safety incidents.
The website takes you through the reporting system.
You can use the NRLS health service eForm to report a patient safety incident if you work in the NHS and the patient involved in the incident was being cared for by the NHS in England or Wales.
Members of the public can make a complaint or report a problem by calling the NPSA on 0207 927 9500 or they can fill in the online reporting form.

Activity 1.5

Go to www.npsa.nhs.uk/advice and list some of the safer practice notices that appear on that website and think of ways in which they may be able to help you provide safer care for the people you care for.

You may have noticed safer practice notices related to:
- Blood transfusions
- Patient identification
- Issues associated with medications
- Equipment, i.e. infusion devices

Activity 1.6

When you are next in a clinical or care area, take the time to find out what type of documentation is used to report issues that concern patient safety. Have a look at the content of the document and find out what it contains, what information is required, and what then happens to the document once it has been completed.

The document may be called different things in different areas; some organisations may call it an accident form and others may refer to it as an incident form. The content of the document, what data and information are required, may also vary from establishment to establishment. You will notice that the person filling in the documentation will need to provide a range of data and information related to the patient safety issue; this must be factual information and, when appropriate, supporting evidence may be required, for example supporting statements from other people involved in the incident.

Activity 1.7

Find out where the following policies are kept in the clinical or care area where you are working:

- Standard (universal) infection control precautions
- Aseptic technique
- Isolation of patients

What is the review date?

The storage of polices and protocols should be easily accessible by all staff, patients and the public so that they can consult them as and when required. Each policy must be clearly marked with a review date (DH, 2006b). There should be an audit trail that will demonstrate compliance with the policy. When new members of staff begin employment with the NHS organisation, information on the policies should be included in the induction programme.

Activity 1.8

Check the policy and procedure in your place of work that is related to the safe disposal of clinical waste. What does it say about the colour of bags to be used for certain categories of waste? Is there only one type of sharps bin in the care area; what other types are there; what are they to be used for?

The storage of polices and protocols should be easily accessible by all staff, patients and the public so that they can consult them as and when required. Each policy must be clearly marked with a review date (DH, 2006b). There should be audit trail that will demonstrate compliance with the policy. When new members of staff begin employment with the NHS organisation, information on the policies should be included in the induction programme.
The different coloured bags are related to the correct segregation of waste:

- Yellow bags are for known hazardous waste, and disposal is by incineration, for example waste contaminated with blood.
- Orange bags are for hazardous waste, for example heavily contaminated incontinence pads, dressing packs if heavily soiled.
- Black bags are for domestic waste, for example mouth pieces from peak flow meters, office waste.

The different coloured sharps bins are related to the correct segregation of waste:

- Yellow lidded sharps bin are for known hazardous sharps and disposal is by incineration, for example disposable needles.
- Orange lidded sharps bins are for hazardous sharps, for example intravenous lines.
- Purple lidded sharps bins are for cytotoxic and cytostatic waste, for example syringes either fully or partially discharged that have contained drugs that are classified as cytotoxic and cytostatic (including vaccines).

Activity 1.9

What PPE is available where you work; do you know how to access it and do you know how to use it?

You may have identified gloves, aprons and face protection (including goggles and masks).

Activity 1.10

Where in your place of work are disinfectant hand rubs available? What do hand hygiene posters in your care area say — what message are they trying to get across?

Hand rubs in hospital settings should be available at every bedside; you may also have seen them at entrances and exits to wards and departments.
Hand hygiene posters aim to encourage hand hygiene for all.

Activity 1.11

With your colleagues' permission watch them clean their hands using either soap and water or disinfectant hand rub, and observe their technique during the procedure. As the process progresses, note if they have completed each of the steps below. If a step is not done properly, take notes on what you have seen. Then ask your colleagues to watch you and do the same activity. Discuss what you all have observed and compare notes.

Step	Completed?	Notes/observation
Palms and backs of hands	Yes/No	
Between fingers	Yes/No	
Nails	Yes/No	
Thumbs	Yes/No	
Fingertips	Yes/No	
Wrists	Yes/No	

Activity 1.12

The results of a back injury can impact on various aspects of an individual's life. See if you can describe what impact may occur on the five aspects of life outlined in this table as a result of a back injury.

Aspect of life	Impact
Financial	Whilst off sick with back injury, salary will still be paid but, if a person is dependent upon earning money through overtime for example, this can impinge on a person's life
Social	Socially, as a result of the back injury a person may not be able to get about as much as they may have done; they may not, for example, be able to get to the gym to meet friends and take part in social activities
Domestic	It may be difficult to carry out daily household chores, for example cleaning or reaching up for things on a higher shelf or conversely bending down to pick things up
Professional	The result of the injury may mean that the person has to seek alternative employment
Family life	A person may not be able to take part in usual family life activities such as picking up and cuddling a child or driving to escort an elderly relative for hospital appointments

Activity 1.13

See if you can find evidence of the TILEO framework at use in your work place.

Was the framework readily available? Was there one?

Activity 1.14 Reflection

Take some time when in clinical practice to reflect on the issue of patient safety; choose an activity that you can use to reflect upon. In the box below write what happened, how you felt, and what you would do differently (if anything) next time you are involved in the promotion of patient safety:

What happened?
● Describe the scenario briefly relating to your learning need

How did it make you feel?
● Did you feel good or bad about it?
● What was good or bad about the situation?
● Did you have adequate underpinning knowledge to carry out the care?
● If you had previous experience of similar situation, was it useful this time?

What would you do differently (if anything) next time?
● Has this personal experience prepared you to do further reading and gained more practice under supervision

This is only a guide. Please address the sub-headings to meet your own learning needs.

References

Barber, N. (2001) Ensuring patients' satisfaction with information about their medications. *Quarterly Health Care* **10** (3), 130–131.

Department of Health (2000) *An Organisation with a Memory* (London: The Stationery Office).

Department of Health (2006a) *Safety First. A Report for Patients, Clinicians and Healthcare Managers* (London: DH).

Department of Health (2006b) *The Code of Practice for the Prevention and Control of Healthcare Associated Infections* (London: DH).

Gould, D. and Drey, N. (2008) Hand hygiene technique. *Nursing Standard* **22** (3), 42–46.

Gould, D., Hewitt-Taylor, J., Drey, N.S., Gammon, J., Chudleigh, J. and Weinberg, J.R. (2007) The clean your hands campaign: critiquing policy and evidence base. *Journal of Hospital Infection* **65** (2), 95–101.

Harriss, A. and Cook, M. (2008) Promoting safe practice. In *Common Foundation Studies in Nursing*, 4th edn, J. Spouse, M. Cook and C. Cox, eds (Edinburgh: Churchill Livingstone), pp. 410–435.

Health and Safety Executive (HSE) (2002) *Handling Home Care: Achieving Safe, Effective and Positive Outcomes for Care Workers and Clients* (London: HSE).

National Patient Safety Agency (NPSA) (2004a) *Seven Steps to Patient Safety. The Full Reference Guide* (London: NPSA).

National Patient Safety Agency (NPSA) (2004b) *Delivering Safer Health Care* (London: NPSA).

Nursing and Midwifery Council (NMC) (2008) *The Code. Standards of Conduct, Performance and Ethics for Nurses and Midwives* (London: NMC).

Parboteeah, S. (2002) Safety in practice. In *Foundations of Nursing Practice: Making the Difference,* 2nd edn, R. Hogston and P.M. Simpson, eds. (Basingstoke: Palgrave), pp. 55–103.

Peate, I. (2008) Body fluids Part 1: infection control. *British Journal of Healthcare Assistants* **2** (1), 6–10.

Pittet, D., Hugonnet, S., Harbarth, S., Mourouga, P., Sauvan, V., Touveneau, S., *et al.* (2000) Effectiveness of a hospital-wide programme to improve compliance with hand hygiene. *The Lancet* **356** (9238), 1307–1312.

Rennie-Meyer, K. (2007) Preventing the spread of infection. In *Foundations of Nursing Practice: Fundamentals of Holistic Care,* C. Brooker and A. Waugh, eds (London: Mosby), pp. 391–423.

Vincent, C. and Coulter, A. (2002) Patient safety: what about the patient? *Quality and Safety in Health Care* **11** (76), 76–80.

Wilson, J. (2006) *Infection Control in Clinical Practice,* 3rd edn (London: Bailliere Tindall).

Further reading

Royal College of Nursing (RCN) (1999) *Guide to the Handling of Patients,* 4th edn (London: RCN).

Useful websites

Department of Health: www.dh.gov.uk

Infection control e-learning programme for NHS staff: http://www.infectioncontrol.nhs.uk/

Healthcare Commission England: www.healthcarecommission.org.uk

Health and Safety Executive: http://www.hse.gov.uk/

National Patient Safety Agency: www.npsa.nhs.uk

National Resource for Infection Control: www.nric.org.uk

2 Principles of medicines management

IAN PEATE

> ## Aims

The aim of this chapter is to introduce you to the key principles associated with the safe administration of medicines and provide you with an overview of the calculation and routes for administering medication.

> ## Learning objectives

On completion of this chapter, you will learn to:
- Understand the importance of administering medicines in a competent and safe manner
- Describe the various routes used for the administration of medicines
- Outline the nursing care required when administering medicines via the various routes
- Describe how the law provides for the safe storage, dispensing and administration of various types of medicines
- Appreciate the need for effective communication
- Demonstrate basic mathematical calculations associated with the safe and effective administration of medicines

Introduction

The administration of medicines is an important aspect of the role and function of the nurse. The Nursing and Midwifery Council (NMC) (NMC, 2008a) state that medicines management should not be seen as a mechanistic task, it requires the nurse to make complex decisions executing their professional judgement.

The safe and effective administration and management of medicines demands that the nurse possesses the necessary knowledge, skills and attitudes; the learner nurse must develop the competence to ensure that the person receiving the medication comes to no harm. The knowledge and skills required for the safe administration of medicines includes an understanding of pharmacology and the biological sciences. This chapter addresses the important prerequisite of numerical competency and effective communication, the theory that underpins and supports the nurse when administering medicines, and a general discussion concerning medicine management.

There are many issues or factors that control or govern the administration of medicines, some of these have been identified above; one other important issue that needs to be given consideration is the legal or statutory aspects associated with medicines. A brief overview of the law and the legal considerations is provided.

A key aspect of the role and function of the nurse is the safe and effective administration of medicines. The nurse administers medicine of various types, for various reasons, to various people via various routes. All pre-registration nursing programmes of study are required to teach about the administration of medicines.

Before you read any further, it should be noted that there are various terms/words used by people, which they use to describe medicines. Can you list the names they might use to describe medicines? Try asking a number of people, ask different people about the words they use to describe medicines, ask young and old people, people from different cultures, sick and well people?

➤ Activity 2.1 Key terms

Using a nursing or medical dictionary or any other resource you think may help you; begin this chapter by finding out the meaning of the words below. You might want to make use of the human resources around you, for example registered nurses, pharmacist or doctor. There are blank spaces provided for you to enter your responses.

Term	Definition
Allergy	
Anaphylaxis	
Balm	
Buccal	
Contraindication	

Activity 2.1 (*Continued*)

Epidural	
Half-life	
Hypodermic	
Hypodermoclysis	
Intradermal	
Transdermal patch	
Intramuscular	
Intraocular	
Intraosseous	
Intravenous	
Lotion	
Ointment	
Pessary	
Subcutaneous	
Sublingual	
Suppository	
Intra-aural	
Intra-vesicular	
Suspension	
Solution	
Cream	
Capsule	
Tablet	
Enema	
Syrup	
Elixir	
Nebuliser	
Inhaler	

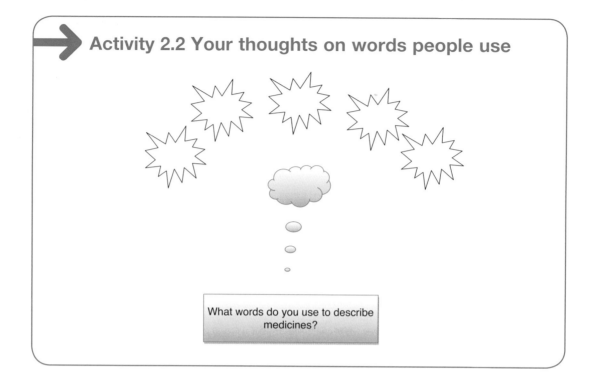

Activity 2.2 Your thoughts on words people use

What words do you use to describe medicines?

One of the words used to describe medicines might have been drugs. The word 'drugs' (depending on who you ask) can mean different things to different people; sometimes, the word is associated with illicit substances. As your list will have shown medicinal products can be defined in many ways, so what is a medicine?

It should be noted that when you administer a prescribed drug to a person (under supervision), the key aim maybe to do the patient good but there may also be side effects associated with some medicines that could result in harm to the person. Although all nursing interventions have the potential to help and also harm the person, the intention is to minimise the potential harm or side effects.

Prescribing and dispensing — an overview

The prescribing and dispensing of medicines are dealt with by a number of government agencies and various professional bodies. These various agencies may be concerned with the licensing and manufacture of medicines for humans. The pharmacist is an invaluable resource if the nurse needs to substantiate or validate a prescription and its contents, but there are others who maybe just as resourceful, for example a doctor.

Prescribing

There are a number of people who can legally prescribe medications and there are several mechanisms that are available for the prescribing of medicines (Modernisation Agency, 2005). In certain instances after consultation with doctors, pharmacists and other healthcare professionals on the list of registered healthcare professionals below can, so long as they stay within the boundaries of the law, prescribe medications using a patient group directive. These could be:

- Nurses
- Paramedics
- Optometrists
- Chiropodists
- Radiographers
- Orthoptists
- Physiotherapists
- Pharmacists
- Dieticians
- Occupational therapists
- Prosthetists and orthoptists
- Speech and language therapists

All of the healthcare professionals mentioned above must be deemed competent, appropriately qualified and educated to use a patient group directive. Can you think of any more?

Dispensing

There are fewer errors associated with the dispensing of medications than there are with the prescribing of them (DH, 2004b). There are exceptional circumstances when nurses may dispense drugs, and when this does occur this must be done in line with local policy and procedure. The dispensing of drugs in some areas is seen as the nurse's extended role; if this is the case, the nurse must practise this activity under the directions of an approved practitioner (DH, 2004b). Members of the general public have a right to know that the nurse who does undertake to dispense will carry out this duty with the same reasonable skill they would expect of a pharmacist.

The administration of medicines — the role of the student

Standard 18 of NMC (2008a) states that 'students must never administer/supply medicinal products without direct supervision'. As a student nurse, the standards outlined in the NMC's Code of Conduct 2008b) also apply to you. You must, at all times, work only within the level of your understanding and competence and always under the direct supervision of a registered nurse or midwife (NMC 2002). This requirement also applies during the administration of medicines or whilst you are assisting with the administration of medicines. You are responsible for your actions or omissions as a student. However, as you are not yet registered with the NMC, you cannot be answerable to them; the registered nurse or midwife who is supervising your practice is ultimately accountable for your actions or omissions. Students must never administer medicines without direct supervision. However, in order to achieve the outcomes and standards required for registration, students must be given opportunities to participate in the administration of medication but this must always be under direct supervision (NMC, 2008a). Nevertheless, you must not forget that you are, and may be, required to be answerable to your educational institution's policies, procedures and rules. You must remain accountable for your actions or omissions in law at all times, just as every other citizen is required to.

The NMC (2002) make clear that as a student you should not participate in any procedure for which you have not been fully prepared or in which you are not being adequately supervised. If you ever find yourself in this position, then you must make this known to your supervisor as quickly as possible. You must always work within the policies and procedures that apply in the area of care where you are working, as well as the advice that has been provided by your educational institution. You may need to access additional sources of information and references, if necessary.

What is a medicine?

The boundaries between medicines and other products are becoming increasingly blurred and this can present problems for those who regulate the control of medicines and those who administer them. Under the Medicines Act 1968, a medicine is defined as 'any substance or combination of substances which may be administered to human beings or animals with a view to making a diagnosis or to restoring, correcting or modifying physiological functions in human beings or animals'.

There are also appliances, instruments and devices that are classed not as medicines but as medical devices. These appliances are also a part of the Act. The range of products varies from syringes and dressings, surgical stockings to surgical instruments, hospital beds and cots and walking frames and even condoms and contact lenses.

Products such as food substances, cosmetics and disinfectants are not usually seen as medicines despite the fact that they may be marketed as being able to 'fight' a disease or 'protect' a person from a disease; these products are not normally required to have a licence. Products such as food supplements that contain additives, for instance minerals or vitamins, are usually subjected to regulations cited in food and safety and labelling legislation.

If, however, a product contains pharmacologically active substances or when it uses marketing and it is stated that it can, for example, reduce cholesterol, then it may be required to have a licence prior to it being released onto the market for sale and purchase by the general public. The licence attempts to ensure that the product is above all safe and effective; a product licence is granted once the product has passed all tests. The granting of the product licence means that it can be used in the treatment of specific medical conditions.

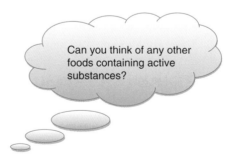

Can you think of any other foods containing active substances?

It can be seen that the term 'medicine' can encompass a range of therapeutic products. It is important that the nurse understands what these products are and how to store and administer them, as well as caring for people receiving medications.

The law

There are a number of elements of legislation that govern the administration of medicines within the UK:

- The Medicines Act 1968
- The Misuse of Drugs Act 1971

There are other legislative points that are also important but not discussed here, for example the various European directives. The Health and Safety at Work Act 1974 is another aspect of legislation that impinges on issues associated with medications; the Act brings much weight to the manufacturing, dispensing, storing and administration of medicines.

The control and regulation of drugs

In this section, legislation will be briefly outlined in order to remind the nurse that there are legal issues associated with drug administration. What also needs to be considered carefully are the various local policies and procedures that must be taken into account; sometimes, these are also referred to as protocols. NHS Trusts, voluntary organisations and the independent healthcare sector will have developed local regulations that govern the administration of medicines; these are sometimes known as policies, procedures and protocols. Standard operating procedures are procedures that have been formulated by organisations to address issues associated with the management of controlled drugs. The policies and procedures formulated must by law comply with the legal regulations that are provided nationally, and in the case of the European directives, internationally.

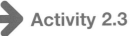 **Activity 2.3**

The next time you are working with a registered nurse, ask about the standard operating procedures that are in place in that organisation that are associated with controlled drugs. Take the time to access those standard operating procedures and make notes below, highlighting the key points.

The Medicines Act 1968

The Medicines Act 1968 brought together most of the previous legislation that related to medicines and initiated a number of other legal provisions for the control of medicines. This Act did not deal with dangerous drugs, in particular; nevertheless many of the requirements of the Act applied to dangerous drugs.

Table 2.1   The three categories created by the Medicines Act 1968

Category	Explanation
Prescription only medicines (POMs)	These medicines may be sold or supplied to the public only on an appropriate practitioner's prescription. They maybe administered only by or in accordance with directions from an appropriate practitioner. With the exception of certain controlled drugs and certain strengths, all controlled drugs are prescription only medicines
Pharmacy medicines (Ps)	Pharmacy medicines are subject to certain exceptions; they maybe sold or supplied only from registered premises by, or under the supervision of, a pharmacist
General sales list medicines (GSLs)	These medicines may be sold or supplied direct to the public in an unopened manufacturer's pack from any lockable premises, often retail outlets. These medicines need neither a prescription nor the supervision of a pharmacist

Medicinal drugs were divided into three categories by this Act; the divisions took into consideration the dangers (or potential dangers) and the risk of misuse. Table 2.1 outlines the three categories.

The Misuse of Drugs Act 1971

The misuse of illegal drugs is a major public health, criminal and social problem (House of Commons, 2006). The possession, storage and destruction of controlled dugs are governed by the Misuse of Drugs Act 1971 as well as other regulations such as the Misuses of Drugs Regulations 2001 (and subsequent amendments). The purpose of the Misuse of Drugs Act 1971 was to provide a coherent framework for drug regulation which prior to this Act was covered by a number of other Acts.

Under the Misuse of Drugs Act 1971, it is an offence to possess a controlled drug unlawfully, to posses drugs with intent to supply, or offer to supply a controlled drug, to allow premises to be used for the purpose of drug taking and to traffic in drugs. Nurses and doctors who possess, supply and give controlled drugs must act within the law; otherwise, they may face prosecution under the Act. For this reason, there are many regulations that govern the use of controlled drugs.

Activity 2.4

When you are next in a clinical area, take some time to find out about the rules and regulations in that area which govern the possession, supply and administration of controlled drugs. Make some notes.

The Misuse of Drugs Regulations 2001 is concerned with the therapeutic use of drugs. These regulations define who the people are who are authorised to supply and possess controlled drugs while acting in their professional capacities; the regulations lay down conditions under which these activities are to be carried out.

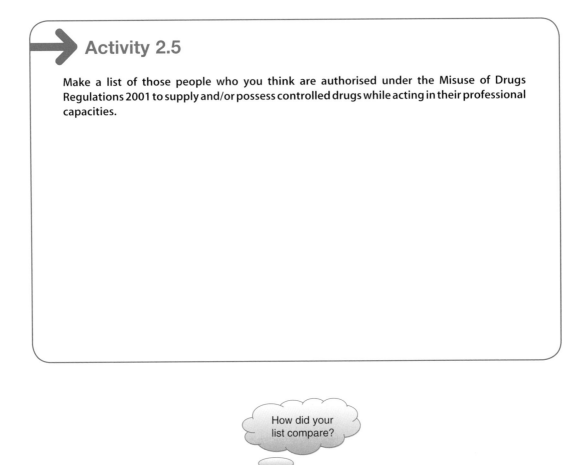

Activity 2.5

Make a list of those people who you think are authorised under the Misuse of Drugs Regulations 2001 to supply and/or possess controlled drugs while acting in their professional capacities.

How did your list compare?

Controlled drugs

The Misuse of Drugs Act 1971 introduced the concept of controlled drugs. Controlled drugs play a vital part in the management of a number of clinical conditions. They are, however, subjected to various legislative controls because they have the potential to be abused or diverted and cause harm (DH, 2006a).

The ABC classification of drugs

Controlled drugs are subjected to special legislative controls (Ahmed and Majeed, 2007). The origin of the ABC classification of drugs has its origins in Misuse of Drugs Act 1971. The ABC classification of drugs system was designed to make it possible to control certain drugs related to their comparative harmfulness to either individuals or to society as a whole when they were misused.

Activity 2.6

Below is a list of drugs that fall under the ABC classificatory system. See if you can arrange them in their classificatory order, where class A drugs are said to cause most risk and carry heavier penalties for possession and supply.

Ecstasy	Gamma-hydroxybutyrate (GHB)	Methylphenidate (Ritalin)
Methyl amphetamine	Anabolic steroids	Barbiturate
Codeine	Crack cocaine	Magic mushrooms
LSD	Amphetamines	Temazepam
Barbiturates	Cocaine	Cannabis
Heroin	Amphetamines (for injection)	Diazepam

Ketamine

Class	Drugs
A	
B	
C	

The current classificatory system (the ABC system) is being reviewed, so changes might occur. It is important with all drugs to keep yourself up to date with changes.

A registered midwife may legally possess in her or his own right the following controlled drugs:

- Diamorphine
- Morphine
- Pethidine
- Pentazocine

The midwife can only possess these controlled drugs as is necessary for the practice of his or her profession. When a midwife invokes this right to posses such controlled drugs, there are strict regulations and protocols that must be adhered to.

Storage of controlled drugs

The aspect of legislation that deals with the safe storage of controlled drugs is The Misuse of Drugs (Safe Custody) Regulations 1973 and addresses, as the name of the legislation suggests, the safe custody of controlled drugs when in certain specified premises (i.e. a hospital ward). These regulations are very detailed with regard to the standards that are required for safes and cabinets that are used in the storage of controlled drugs. Cupboards must conform to the British Standard reference BS2881 or otherwise approved by the pharmacy department.

Below are some key points that should be taken into account when storing controlled drugs in hospital wards:

- When cupboards that are used for the storage of controlled drugs are in use, they must be kept locked.
- The lock that is used for the storage of controlled drugs must not be common to any other lock in the hospital.
- Keys must only be made available to authorised members of staff.
- The cupboard must only be used for the storage of controlled drugs. No other medicines or items are allowed to be stored in the cupboard used for controlled drugs.
- All controlled drug must be locked away when not in use.

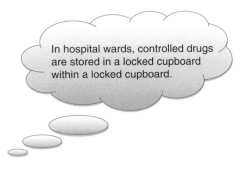

In hospital wards, controlled drugs are stored in a locked cupboard within a locked cupboard.

Mathematics and the administration of medicines

Woodrow (1998) points out that people do not become nurses to practise mathematics. However, all nurses must have an understanding of calculus if they are to perform their job effectively and above all, safely. Hence, it is important that nurses are able to carry out accurate drug calculations and other arithmetically based activities to perform within the realms of the code of professional conduct (NMC, 2008b) — doing the patient no harm and acting in their best interests, drug calculations are an essential skill (Wright, 2004). The use of calculus is predominantly associated with the administration of drugs but not exclusively with the administration of drugs.

Hutton (2005) suggests that the nurse should apply common sense rules to drug calculations, for example, what a sensible answer should be. Knowing what should be a sensible answer comes with experience; however, the nurse should never make assumptions. It should never be assumed that the prescription is correct and if in doubt referral to recommended dose ranges published in drug formularies is needed.

The nurse's ability to calculate accurately can be flawed. Trim (2004) highlights that over the last decade discrepancies associated with the nurse's competence to calculate correctly have been noted. Errors are associated with incorrect calculations occurring in all branches of nursing, and within all areas of nursing, these errors have the potential to threaten the lives and well-being of the people nurses care for (Gray and Jackson, 2004; Weeks et al., 2000). The mathematical calculations that nurses are required to deal with, such as calculating drug doses, are becoming more critical and complex (Weeks et al., 2000). Therefore, it is vital that nurses regularly update and continue to develop their skills in association with drug calculations. The NMC (2008a) state that use of calculators to determine the volume or quantity of medication should not act as a substitute for arithmetical knowledge and skill.

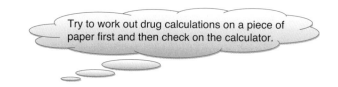

Try to work out drug calculations on a piece of paper first and then check on the calculator.

This chapter cannot address every mathematical problem that you may face; it provides a basic introduction to simple mathematical calculations and the application to practice. You are advised to hone your numeracy skills whenever the opportunity arises; there are several ways in which you can do this, for example, by using both human and material resources. At every stage of the calculation process, should you feel unsure or in doubt, you must seek help, advice and support. The following points may help you in the clinical area to ensure safe practice:

- The patient's best interests come first.
- Work out calculations in a quiet area, take your time.
- Recheck and ask a colleague to examine what you have done if you think the answer looks unusual.
- Use a calculator and other aids if you need to.
- If you are still unsure, do not give the drug; seek help.

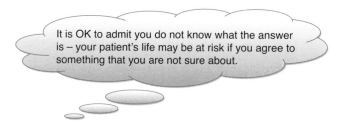

It is OK to admit you do not know what the answer is – your patient's life may be at risk if you agree to something that you are not sure about.

In the UK, the predominant system of measurement (in healthcare) is the metric system SI — Le Systeme International d'Unites (SI). Common decimal weights are listed in the box below.

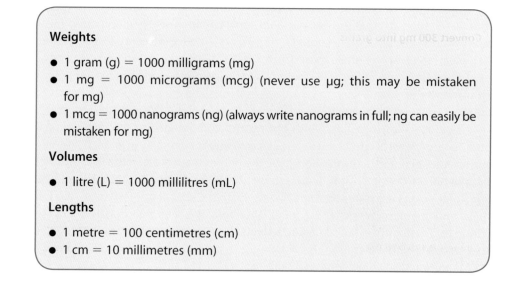

Weights

- 1 gram (g) = 1000 milligrams (mg)
- 1 mg = 1000 micrograms (mcg) (never use μg; this may be mistaken for mg)
- 1 mcg = 1000 nanograms (ng) (always write nanograms in full; ng can easily be mistaken for mg)

Volumes

- 1 litre (L) = 1000 millilitres (mL)

Lengths

- 1 metre = 100 centimetres (cm)
- 1 cm = 10 millimetres (mm)

Table 2.2   Numbers in words and figures

Numbers in words	Numbers in figures			
	Thousands	Hundreds	Tens	Units
Two hundred and fifty-eight	—	2	5	8
Six thousand four hundred	6	4	0	0
Eighty-nine	—	—	8	9
Twenty-one	—	—	2	1

Note: Milligrams and millilitres are plural as are metres, centimetres and millimetres; however, the appropriate abbreviations are:

mg **NOT** mgs and mL **NOT** mLs, m **NOT** ms, cm **NOT** cms and mm **NOT** mms.

Place value is associated with numbers, and where each number from 0 to 9 is written in a column, for example:

- Units
- Tens
- Hundreds
- Thousands

Table 2.2 demonstrates numbers written in words and in figures.

Numbers that are smaller than 1/unit are decimals, for example, tenths, hundredths and thousandths. These are separated by the decimal point, see Figure 2.1.

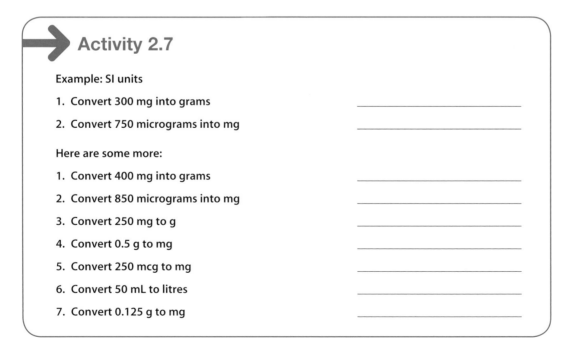

Activity 2.7

Example: SI units

1. Convert 300 mg into grams   _____

2. Convert 750 micrograms into mg   _____

Here are some more:

1. Convert 400 mg into grams   _____

2. Convert 850 micrograms into mg   _____

3. Convert 250 mg to g   _____

4. Convert 0.5 g to mg   _____

5. Convert 250 mcg to mg   _____

6. Convert 50 mL to litres   _____

7. Convert 0.125 g to mg   _____

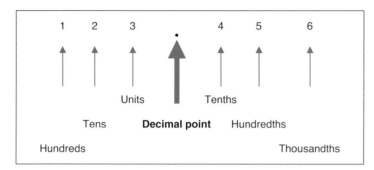

Figure 2.1   Numbers and the decimal point

Adding and subtracting decimals

You will be required to use addition and subtraction nearly every day in your work, for example, when calculating a patient's fluid balance. In most cases of fluid balance, decimal points are not required; you would round up or down to the nearest whole number. However, in the acutely ill or the neonate, for example, exact amounts may be required. In Activity 2.8, calculate the amount of fluid the child has had via the intravenous route for 24 h. Then calculate the amount of fluid aspirated from the nasogastric tube and urine via the urinary catheter. Total the input and output values, subtracting input from output, and arrive at the child's fluid balance; is it negative or positive?

Numbers that are left to the decimal point are greater than 1. Those numbers situated right to the decimal point are less than 1. In the following example, note the position of the decimal point:

1.60 is equal to 1 plus a fraction of 1 (6/10)
0.75 is equal to a fraction of 1 (75/100 or three-quarters)

Multiplying decimals

Often drug calculations require you to multiply and divide. To multiply a decimal is done in exactly the same way as you multiply whole numbers; however, you have to consider the decimal point. Always remember to put the decimal point in the correct place when you arrive at your answer.

When multiplying, you have to use the 'power of ten rule':

× 10 move the decimal point one place to the right
× 100 move the decimal point two places to the right
× 1000 move the decimal point three places to the right

Here is an example:

6.178 × 100 = 617.8

Try this one next:

0.0345 × 10 = 0.345

Activity 2.8 Total the fluid chart

Getwell Hospital
Fluid Balance Chart

Name...
Ward..
Hospital number..
DoB...

Time	Input (in mL)		Output (in mL)		
	Intravenous	Oral/other	Urine	Other	Comments
0000	2.60	NBM	20		
0100	2.65		10	1.20	Nasogastric
0200	2.75		10		
0300	3.84		8.2		
0400	8.70		2.6		
0500	6.00		8.0	1.80	Nasogastric
0600	6.00		12.2		
0700	9.90		10.2		
0800	3.65		10		
0900	7.75		14	1.10	Nasogastric
1000	12.00		13		
1100	12.75		14.7		
1200	20.00		12.4		
1300	21.20		20	1.20	Nasogastric
1400	22.00		32		
1500	75.00		36		
1600	75.00		26		
1700	15.00		28	1.75	Nasogastric
1800	0.75		23		
1900	0.75		22		
2000	1.75		18		
2100	10.75		12.8	1.80	Nasogastric
2200	20.75		14.6		
2300	21.75		12.4		
Total		Nil			

Multiplying by	Number of zeros	Movement of the decimal point to the right
10	1	1 place
100	2	2 places
1000	3	3 places
10 000	4	4 places
Dividing by	Number of zeros	Movement of the decimal point to the left
10	1	1 place
100	2	2 places
1000	3	3 places
10 000	4	4 places

Figure 2.2   Movement of the decimal point in multiplication and division

Division also has the 'power of ten rules'. In multiplication, you move the decimal point to the right, in division it is to the left:

÷ 10 move the decimal point one place to the left
÷ 100 move the decimal point two places to the left
÷ 1000 move the decimal point three places to the left

For example, if dividing 35.42 by 10, 100 and 1000:

÷ 35.42 by 10 = 3.542
÷ 35.42 by 100 = 0.3542
÷ 35.42 by 1000 = 0.03542

Figure 2.2 shows multiplication and division of decimals.

Converting from one unit to another

In some instances, you will be required to convert from one unit to another, for example, from grams to milligrams or from milligrams to micrograms. It is often safer to work in whole numbers, for example, 275 mcg as opposed to 0.275 mg. Fewer mistakes are made when working this way, therefore, being able to convert from one unit to another is required, you need to either multiply or divide. When converting from a larger unit to a smaller unit, multiply by 1000. When converting from a smaller unit to a larger unit, divide by 1000.

Converting 4 g to milligrams, for example (a larger unit to a smaller unit), requires you to multiply by 1000 (1 g = 1000 mg); 4 g in milligrams is equal to 4000 mg. If you were required to convert 10 kg to grams (recall 1 kg = 1000 g):

10 × 1000 = 10 000 g

Activity 2.9

The above are being converted from a larger unit to a smaller unit. Consider now how you would convert from a smaller unit to a larger unit, 3300 mg to grams. You need to divide:

3300 ÷ 1000 = 3.3 g

Converting g to mcg requires you to follow two steps. Convert g to mg, and then convert mg to mcg.

For example, convert 3.5 g to mcg.

3.5 × 1000 = 3500 mg

3500 mg × 1000 = 3 500 000 mcg

Table 2.3   Some forms of medicines

| How much/how many tablets | Solid medication, for example, tablets or capsules |
| How much/how many millilitres | Injections |

The above examples are easier than some real-life challenges you may encounter when working in the clinical field. You must refer to other sources for more detailed explanations of the above, as well as follow the examples that are being provided to you.

All calculations can be written as equations and this will now be demonstrated. There are several formulae that can be used to calculate drug dosages. Formulae consist of ratios to set proportions, and can be used to calculate dosages for solid and liquid preparations. The standard formula for calculating drug dosage is related to the form of medication the patient is to receive (see Table 2.3).

The formula that applies to all of the above is:

$$\text{Volume required} = \frac{\text{Strength required}}{\text{Stock strength}}$$

Or

$$\frac{\text{What you want}}{\text{What you have}} \quad \frac{(X)}{(\text{what it's in})}$$

For example, a patient has been prescribed 75 mg of pethidine intramuscular injection. The stock you have comes in ampoules of 100 mg in 1 mL.

$$\text{Volume required} = \frac{\text{Strength required (75 mg)}}{\text{Stock strength (100 mg)}}$$

$$\frac{75}{100} \times 1\,\text{mL}$$

$$= \frac{75}{100} \times \frac{1}{1}$$

$$= 0.75\,\text{mL}$$

Another example, a patient is prescribed 225 mg of ranitidine orally. The medication comes in 150 mg tablets.

$$\text{Volume required} = \frac{\text{Strength required (225 mg)}}{\text{Stock strength (150 mg)}}$$

$$\frac{225}{150} \times 1$$

$$= 1.5 \text{ (or one and a half tablets)}$$

Example. A patient is prescribed 1.5 g of Flucloxacillin, stock available is 750 mg tablets. The prescribed amount and the available stock must be in the same units.

Convert grams to milligrams

- 1.5 g is the same as 1500 mg

- $$\frac{1500 \text{ mg}}{750 \text{ mg}} = 2$$

Activity 2.10

1. If a patient requires 20 mg and each tablet is 5 mg, how many tablets are required?

2. A patient is prescribed 1.5 g of Flucloxacillin; stock available is 750 mg capsules. How many capsules does the patient require?

3. A patient is prescribed 120 mg of Frusemide; the tablets available are 40 mg. How many tablets are required?

4. A 50 mg dose is prescribed; tablets are 12.5 mg each. How many tablets will you give?

5. A 625 mg dose is prescribed; tablets are 1.25 g each. How many tablets will you give?

6. A 150 mg dose is prescribed; tablets are 50 mg each. How many tablets will you give?

7. A 75 mg dose is prescribed; tablets are 25 mg each. How many tablets would you give?

8. A 25 mg dose is prescribed; tablets are 12.5 mg each. How many tablets would you give?

9. A 1 mg dose is prescribed; tablets are 500 micrograms each. How many tablets will you give?

10. Three tablets each contain 250 mg. What is the total dose in milligrams?

Principles for underpinning the practice of administration of medicines

The Standards for Medicines (NMC, 2008a) are provided to practitioners in the form of guidance; they are not rules to be strictly adhered to but are merely guiding principles that should be used in conjunction with sound clinical judgement and in accordance to local policies. The standards outlined by the NMC (2008a) are minimum standards and should be used to provide you with a benchmark by which your practice should be measured. The standards do not provide you with guidance that will cover every single situation that you may come across during practice (and neither will the contents of this chapter); the purpose is to encourage the thinking through of issues and applying professional expertise and judgement, with the best interests of the patient first and foremost.

The first prerequisite for the safe and effective administration of medicines is knowledge and understanding about drugs (types, dose), their proposed actions, drug interactions, their potential side effects. It is vital that prior to administering any drug a sound understanding of that drug is required. A good pharmacology text is essential as well as learning to use publications such as the British National Formulary (BNF).

➤ Activity 2.11

There are no answers to this activity as you have been asked to use the British National Formulary to learn how to use that publication and also to learn about the various medicines, the comments here are prompts

Drug	Generic and/or propriety name	Adult dose	Route(s) of admini- stration	Contra- indications	Side effects	Category

Checking the prescription

The prescription (or a direction to supply) must be checked prior to administering any medicine. The registered nurse must check that the prescription:

- is not for a substance to which the patient is allergic or otherwise unable to tolerate;
- is based, wherever possible, on the patient's informed consent and awareness of the purpose of the treatment;
- is clearly written, typed or computer generated and indelible;
- specifies the substance to be administered, using its generic or brand name where appropriate and its stated form, together with the strength, dosage, timing, frequency of administration, start and finish dates and routes of administration;
- is signed and dated by the authorised prescriber;
- in the case of controlled drugs, specifies the dosage and the number of dosage units or total course, and is signed and dated by the prescriber using relevant documentation as introduced.

The registered nurse must ensure that he/she has:

- clearly identified the patient for whom the medication is intended;
- recorded the weight of the patient on the prescription sheet for all children, and where the dosage of medication is related to weight or surface area (e.g. cytoxic medications) or where clinical condition dictates recorded the patient's weight.

Administration of medicines

The NMC (2008a) provide detailed guidance in relation to medicines management. These standards must be adhered to in conjunction with local trust policies, protocols and procedures; your university or college may have also issued you with guidance. Once the prescription has been checked and the medicinal product that has been prescribed is appropriate for the patient, the medication can be administered. The registered nurse (or the student nurse under supervision) in acting in the best interest of the patient must:

- be certain of the identity of the patient to whom the medicine is to be administered;
- check that the patient is not allergic to the medicine prior to administering it;
- know the therapeutic uses of the medicine to be administered, its normal dosage, side effects, precautions and contraindications;
- be aware of the patient's plan of care;
- check that the prescription or the label on the medicine dispensed is clearly written and unambiguous;
- check the expiry date (where it exists) of the medicine to be administered;
- have considered the dosage, weight where appropriate, method of administration, route and timing;
- administer or withhold in the context of the patient's condition (e.g. the drug digoxin should not normally be administered if the patient's pulse is below 60 beats per minute) and coexisting therapies, for example physiotherapy;

- contact the prescriber or another authorised prescriber without delay whe...
  the prescribed medicine are discovered, where the patient develops a reacti...
  or where assessment of the patient indicates that the medicine is no longer suit...
- make clear, accurate and immediate record of all medicines administered,
  withheld or refused by the patient, ensuring the signature is clear and legible; it...
  responsibility of the registered nurse to ensure that a record is made when delegating...
  of administering medicine (e.g. to a student nurse);
- record the reason for not giving medication.

Griffith *et al.* (2003) discuss the safe administration of medicines. They state that there are five Rs that the nurse must take into consideration in order to ensure that medicines are administered safely and effectively. Table 2.4 considers six Rs, not just the five, as suggested by Griffith *et al.* (2003).

Table 2.4   The six Rs and administration of medicines
(*Source:* Adapted from Griffith *et al.* (2003)).

Right patient	The identity of the patient must be checked; you must be certain of the identity of the patient to whom the medicine is to be administered. Name bands are often used to do this. If in doubt, ask the patient his or her name. Where there are difficulties in clarifying an individual's identity, for example, in some areas of learning disabilities, patients with dementia or confusional states, an up-to-date photograph should be attached to the prescription chart. Check the name and hospital number against the patient's wristband and prescription chart.
Right medicine	Prescriptions must be written in a clear and unambiguous manner. The label on the medicine must also be clear, easy to read and if appropriate have guidelines that are easy to follow. The nurse must be certain about what is to be dispensed; if there is any doubt then the prescriber must be contacted and the prescription rewritten, the The same is true of the label on medicines, ; any problems should be directed towards the pharmacist. The nurse must check the expiry date of drugs every time they are used.
Right dose	The correct dose must be given to the patient; if the dose is not known or the nurse is not familiar with the dosage then this must be checked using a reliable source. The nurse must check the dose to be given. Administering the correct dose requires numeracy

(*continued*)

ble 2.4   (*Continued*)

	skills. If at any stage of the calculation exercise there is any doubt, do not give the drug. Check with the prescriber and the pharmacist. Take time to make drug calculations and do not be intimidated or coerced into agreeing a calculated dose if you do not agree. Prescriptions must be written out clearly and in full; weight or volume must also be clearly expressed. You must be particularly alert to the decimal point used on the prescription chart, the medicine container and when calculating.
	it is important that the medication is given at the right time. For some types of drugs, therapeutic drug levels need to be maintained. If there is any doubt as to whether a drug has already been given, do not repeat the dose check with appropriate staff concerned and inform the prescriber and if appropriate the pharmacist. Frequency may differ at the request of the prescriber and some drugs must be given at certain times of the day; some must be given with a full stomach and some on an empty stomach.
Right route	This aspect of the six Rs is related to whether the drug is to be given orally, intramuscularly or by some other route. It is important that you note the correct route; some medicines cannot be given via some routes and dosages can differ based on the route of administration.
Right documentation	The sixth R — the right documentation — refers to documenting the medicine administered, withheld or refused on the correct form/chart/sheet. Failure to document correctly can lead to a medication error, for example, the dose may be repeated as there is no record that the initial dose was given.

Drug administration errors

A prescribed medicine is the most common treatment provided for patients in the NHS. General practitioners in England issue more than 600 million prescriptions each year; in hospitals this figure is approximately 200 million DH, 2004a.

Most of the medications that are prescribed and administered in the UK are done so safely; however, there are errors that occur and the effects of these errors can be distressing and the consequences serious for all concerned — the person who has been effected by the error, his or her family, the individual who has prescribed the medicine, the dispenser and the administrator. Medication errors can be referred to as adverse drug events and serious errors are known as serious untoward incidences. Errors that do occur can be prevented. There are a number of reasons why drug errors might occur. Gray and Jackson (2004) suggest that this may be because of the increase in technology and the considerable range of drugs that are available. Failure to follow the correct procedure is a cause of medicine error, however; there are other causes such as workload, shift pattern worked, time of day and environmental factors that can also contribute to the number of errors made in association with the administration of medicines.

If a medication error has occurred, then the registered nurse must ensure that he/she reports the error as soon as possible to the prescriber and the line manager. An open and thorough investigation must take place to determine if any improvements to local practice in the administration of medicinal products can be discussed, identified and disseminated. The need for an open culture with regard to the investigation is vital if the immediate reporting of medication errors is to be encouraged.

Covert administration of medicines

The covert administration of medicines can include the deceptive administration of medicines disguised in food or drink. The issue is complex and involves respecting the patients' autonomy to choose, their informed consent and upholding their rights with respect to the Human Rights Act 1998. Administering medicine in a covert way can be regarded as deception. Administering in a deceptive manner should not be confused with the administration of medicines against an individual's will; in the later case, this may be unlawful.

The overriding principle associated with the covert administration of medicines has to be that the nurse is acting in the patient's best interests. The nurse administering medicine is also accountable for his or her actions. An assessment of risk must be undertaken, and at all stages of the process, it is imperative that up-to-date records are maintained; these records should be able to support and demonstrate a duty of care to the patient.

All Trusts should have policies and protocols in place that will inform the nurse of local action. These protocols and policies should be regularly revised and developed as needed. The NMC NMC, 2006) has provided advice regarding the issue of covert medicine administration.

Routes of administration

There are many routes than can be used to administer medicines; most medicines come in a variety of types or formats, some maybe more effective in one type than another. Some of the routes are chosen for specific reasons, for example, for patient convenience or for efficacy. The route of administration must be clearly stated on the prescription chart. After administration of the medicine, the patient must be monitored to determine if there have been any adverse reactions, and if the medicine has been effective, the outcome must be detailed in the appropriate documentation. Regardless of the route of administration, the nurse must always ensure that he/she administers the medicines in accordance with local policy and procedure. This section of the chapter provides information about some of the routes that may be used in the administration of medicines. The information provided should be seen as the principles underpinning the administration of medicines.

Oral medication

This route of administration, administration by mouth, is the most common route for medicines administration. Oral medications come in variety of forms, for example suspension and tablet. Swallowing whole is important for capsules or some tablets because chewing or breaking them may render them less effective. Most tablets and capsules are best taken with a glass of water to help them go down; it may be that some people need plenty of water to help the medicine go down as the tablet could become lodged in the oesophagus causing irritation.

Some oral medicines are to be taken sublingually, that is, they dissolve under the tongue. The medicine in this form is absorbed very quickly, with the desired effect happening almost immediately (e.g. glyceryl trinitrate (GTN)).

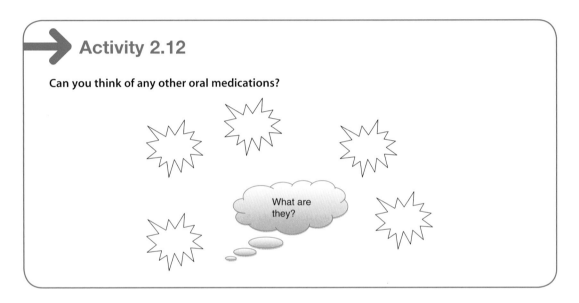

Activity 2.12

Can you think of any other oral medications?

What are they?

All oral medicines come in different strengths. If suspensions are being used to administer the drug then it is important that the suspension is shaken well prior to pouring the suspension on the spoon, into a measuring pot or via the oral syringe. If a medicine pot is being used, the suspension should be prepared upon a flat surface and measuring must take place at eye level to ensure an accurate dose is being given to the patient. If tablets are being used then at all costs the nurse should avoid having to halve or cut the tablet in order to provide the correct dose. If this is necessary then advice from the pharmacist should be sought.

With regard to the crushing or dissolving of medicines, again, this should be avoided as some medicines are unsuitable for crushing (e.g. those with an enteric coating, those for slow or modified release) or dissolving. Slow or modified release medicines are useful when the medicine that has been prescribed has to be slowly released; this way there is a more constant level of the medicine in the blood stream. Soluble or dispersible medicines can be safely dissolved in water, for example soluble aspirin. The advantage of this method of administration is that the medicine can be taken in liquid format; some people find this easier and furthermore it makes the taking of larger tablets easier to swallow.

Crushing of medicines and then administering them via the nasogastric route should be discouraged unless this practice has been deemed safe by the pharmacist. If a patient is unable to swallow tablets, then it may be more appropriate to provide that medicine in the form of a suspension or to consider another route of administration, for example intravenously. At all times during the procedure, the nurse must communicate with the patient explaining about the medicines, being prepared to answer any questions the patient may have and taking the opportunity, if appropriate, to offer health education.

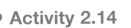

Activity 2.13

When administering oral medications, what equipment is required?

Activity 2.14

Try these oral drug calculations:

1. Patient requires analgesia. He can have Paracetamol Elixir 500 mg. The elixir contains 250 mg in 10 mL. How many millilitres will he require?

2. If a patient required 100 mg and each bottle contains 250 mg in 5 mL, how much do you give?

3. Sodium valporate oral solution is supplied as 200 mg/5 mL. The patient requires 300 mg. How many millilitres does the patient require?

4. If a patient required 250 mg and each bottle contains 125 mg in 5 mL, how much do you give?

5. Linctus is available as 25 mg in 5 mL and we need to give the patient 75 mg. What volume will be given?

Intravenous medication

Intravenous medicines are given directly into the vein. These medicines can be given via a bolus intermittent dose, continuously or intermittent infusion, via a peripheral line or a central line. The choice of the method to be used for drug administration depends upon the treatment. There are advantages and disadvantages associated with intravenous injections.

➡️ ## Activity 2.15

Write here what you think the advantages and disadvantages are associated with intravenous injections.

Advantages	Disadvantages

Intravenous pumps are often used to control the administration of intravenous medications. There are a large number of intravenous pumps available and the nurse must be familiar with their use prior to using them. Quinn (2000) points out that a number of drug errors associated with the use of intravenous pumps and intravenous drug administration occurs as a result of staffs' unfamiliarity with the equipment.

The administration of intravenous medications must only be undertaken by a registered nurse. The registered nurse undertaking the activity must adhere to local requirements, for example, the undertaking of an appropriate Trust assessment training programme and being able to demonstrate competence.

Intramuscular medication

Injections that are directly injected into the muscle are called intramuscular injections. There are number of muscles in which the injection can be given, for example:

- Deltoid muscle — usually used for the administration of small volumes of drugs.
- Quadriceps muscle — often used for IM injections.

● Gluteus maximums muscle — another common site. The injection is given into the upper outer quadrant of the buttock, this site is chosen so as to avoid unintentional damage to the sciatic nerve.

Activity 2.16

Look at these diagrams (see Figure 2.3) and see where the muscles described above are situated?

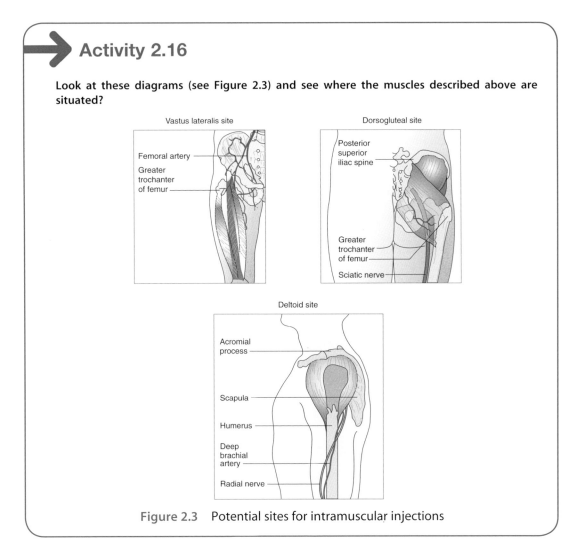

Figure 2.3   Potential sites for intramuscular injections

Injection into the muscle tissue allows for the medication to be absorbed into the systematic circulation; depending on the preparation, this can be either fairly quickly or more slowly. The needle used goes through the skin and into the muscle and the medication is released when the plunger of the syringe is depressed. When the medication has been delivered into the muscle, the needle is safely removed.

The syringe has three major parts:

● The needle
● The barrel
● The plunger

The barrel holds the medicine; the needle goes into the skin and then into the muscle and the plunger is depressed to release the medication into the muscle. Down the side of the barrel are graduated markings relating to millilitres (mL). Medicines to be given via the intramuscular route are always prescribed in millilitres.

Prior to administration, check carefully the prescription sheet and apply the six Rs as described in Table 2.4. Check the vial or ampoule to make sure that it is the right medicine, the right dose and that the drug has not expired. Some medicines that are to be injected need to be reconstituted from a powder into a liquid and the manufacturer's instructions must be followed in order to do this safely. During the preparation stage, ensure that you have washed your hands and that you have plenty of space and light available to prepare and draw up the medication.

When the right amount of drug has been drawn up and you have identified that it is the right patient, the right drug, the right route and the right time, you are now ready to give the drug. All medications administered by student nurses must be administered under the direct supervision of a registered nurse or midwife (NMC, 2008a).

Giving the intramuscular injection

- Wash your hands prior to giving the injection.
- Provide the patient with dignity by ensuring that doors are closed, curtains drawn.
- Explain the procedure to the patient.
- Ensure that there is sufficient lighting and the height of the bed has been adjusted to ensure that you are ergonomically safe.
- Position the patient for the injection, exposing minimal anatomy.
- Put gloves on.
- Clean the site of injection with an alcohol wipe if this is policy using a circular motion.
- Remove the needle guard (sheath) ensuring that the needle only touches the inside of the guard.
- Stretch the skin taut, with the other hand over the injection site.
- Holding the syringe like a dart, then insert the needle into the skin quickly at the correct angle (90°).
- With the other hand, pull back gently on the plunger if no blood is aspirated then inject the medication by pushing the plunger slowly into the barrel with even pressure.

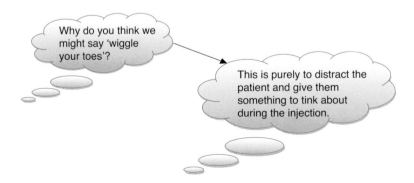

- Steady the patient's tissue that is immediately adjacent to the puncture site with your other hand and quickly remove the needle.

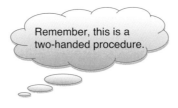

Remember, this is a two-handed procedure.

- If it is policy, gently massage the injection site with an alcohol wipe.
- Lower the bed and leave the patient comfortable.
- Never resheath or replace the needle guard; dispose of the used needle and syringe into the nearest sharps box in accordance with policy.
- Complete all necessary documentation.

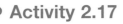

Activity 2.17

Try these drug calculations for injections:
1. A client is ordered 45 mg of Loxapine by intramuscular injection. A 50 mg dose in 1 mL of liquid for IM Injection is available. How many millilitres will you administer?

2. A client is ordered Pethidine 35 mg IM as a pre-medication. Stock ampoules contain 50 mg per mL. What volume must be withdrawn for injection?

3. A client is ordered 100 mg by intramuscular injection. A 50 mg dose in 1 mL of liquid for IM Injection is available. How many millilitres will you administer?

4. A client is ordered 25 mg by intramuscular injection. A 50 mg dose in 1 mL of liquid for IM Injection is available. How many millilitres will you administer?

5. A client is ordered 300 mg by intramuscular injection. A 100 mg dose in 1 mL of liquid for IM Injection is available. How many millilitres will you administer?

Subcutaneous medication

The most common forms of medication administered via the subcutaneous route (injections given under the skin into the subcutaneous tissues) are:

- Insulin
- Anticoagulants
- Analgesia

A syringe with medicine in it is attached to a needle, the medicine is injected into the subcutaneous tissue by pressing the plunger and releasing the medicine, and after this the needle is removed. Common sites for administration of subcutaneous injection are:

- The upper arm
- Anterior aspects of the thighs
- Upper back
- Abdominal wall

A number of factors need to be taken into consideration with regard to subcutaneous injections. The amount of medicine to be injected; this is small when using this route and the medicine is absorbed slowly. The frequency of medication; for example, if anticoagulant therapy is being given regularly, then the site must be rotated; this prevents fibrosis, which may hinder absorption of the medication. Hence, the type of medication can dictate the site to be used. Figure 2.4 outlines some of the sites used in rotating subcutaneous injections.

Prior to administration of the subcutaneous injection, check carefully the prescription sheet and apply the six Rs as described in Table 2.4. Check the vial or ampoule to make sure that it is the right medicine; some subcutaneous medicines come ready prepared in the syringe, which also needs to be checked. Ensure that it is the right dose and that the drug has not expired. Some medicines that are to be injected need to be reconstituted from a powder into a liquid and the manufacturer's instructions must be followed in order to do this safely. During the preparation stage, ensure that you have washed your hands and that you have plenty of space and light available to prepare and draw up the medication.

When the right amount of drug has been drawn up and you have identified that it is the right patient, the right drug, the right route and the right time, you are now ready to give the drug.

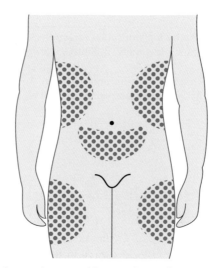

Figure 2.4   Some sites used in rotating subcutaneous injections

Giving the subcutaneous injection

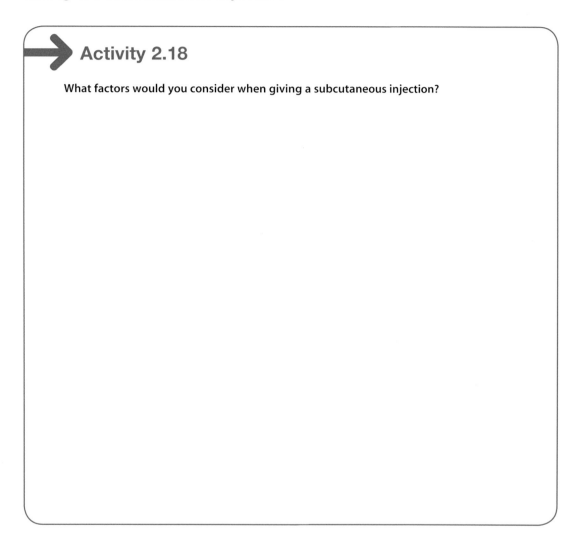

Hypodermoclysis is associated with the insertion of a small cannula (a butterfly cannula) into the subcutaneous tissues (usually this is in the abdomen). The cannula is secured using an occlusive type of dressing and the prescribed infusion begins. The rate and duration of fluid to be transfused is determined by prescription and the care and management of the patient is in accordance with local policy. It is vital that all fluids (input and output) are recorded on the fluid balance chart.

Suppositories

Suppository is one form of rectal medicine; other forms include enema, creams and gels. These are discussed further in chapter 6 With suppository, the medicine is inserted into the rectum and dissolves slowly at body temperature and as it dissolves it is absorbed into the surrounding tissue and the blood stream as there is a rich blood supply in this area. Suppositories are solid bullet-shaped preparations that have been designed for easy insertion into the anus (see Figure 2.5).

How to insert a suppository

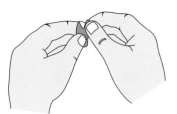

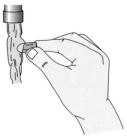

1. Remove foil wrapper.

2. Moisten the suppository with water or water-based lubricating jelly (such as K-Y).

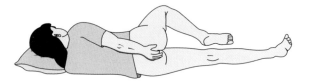

3. Lie on your left side and bend your right knee up towards your chest. Gently push the suppository into your rectum so that it is deep enough not to come out.

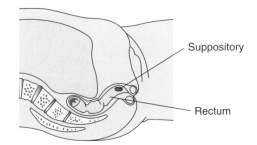

Figure 2.5   How to insert a suppository

This type of medicine dissolves slowly and releases the active ingredient of the medicine. There are a number of reasons why suppositories may be used:

- Not being able to swallow.
- Severe nausea or vomiting.
- The medicine might be destroyed by gastric acids.
- An effect is required locally, for example, the treatment of haemorrhoids, or ulcerative colitis.

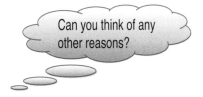

Can you think of any other reasons?

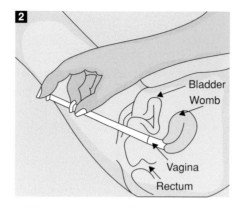

Figure 2.6   Insertion of a pessary

Pessaries

Medicines that are inserted into the vagina are called pessaries. The medication is gradually released into the vagina at body temperature (see Figure 2.6).

Pessaries are solid bullet-shaped preparations that have been designed for easy insertion into the vagina. Pessaries can be inserted with the fingers or by the use of an applicator. As the pessary melts, the medication may leak from the vagina, and the patient may be encouraged to insert the pessary at night prior to going to bed as opposed to during the day. If the pessary is inserted during the day, the woman may be advised to use a sanitary towel to prevent any staining of the clothes.

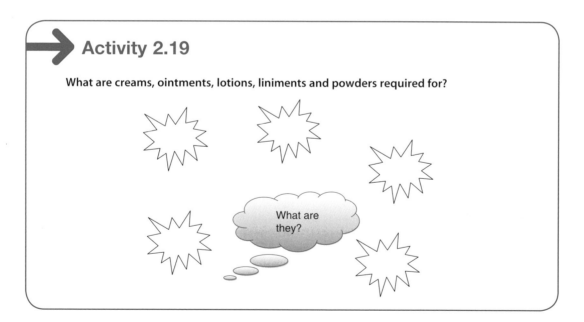

Activity 2.19

What are creams, ointments, lotions, liniments and powders required for?

What are they?

Intraocular medication

Ophthalmic medications are those that are used in the eye.

Activity 2.20

There are several reasons why a person may need to have ophthalmic medications. List below what you think these may be.

Any medications used in the eyes are always sterile. The six Rs described in Table 2.4 must be adhered to when administering eye medication; in addition to this, the nurse has to ensure that the correct eye is being medicated, that is, right or left. Eye medications are often dispensed from dropper top type bottles or if an ointment, in a tube. Medication can be a single-dose package or multi-dose containers. The actual dose of liquid medication must be measured directly into the eye as drops from the bottle. If ointment is being administered, then the dose will be the length of ointment extruded that fits the conjunctival sac (Ellis and Bentz, 2007). At all times, local policy and procedure must be adhered to with regard to the procedure that must be used when instilling eye medications.

Nurse prescribing

There are mechanisms in place that allow for nurses to act as independent prescribers. These mechanisms provide a guide for the prescribing, supplying and administering of medicines (DH, 2006b), and they should be used in conjunction with other sources of information and references.

Independent nurse prescribing allows nurses to prescribe any licensed medicine for any medical condition that a nurse prescriber is competent to treat; this also includes some controlled drugs. In effect, independent nurse prescribing allows the nurse to prescribe any licensed medicine in the BNF to be prescribed.

All first-level registered nurses, midwives and registered specialist community public health nurses may train to be independent prescribers. However, the NMC (2005) demand that those nurses and midwives who wish to become independent practitioners must have at least 3 years post-registration experience.

The thrust behind the development and implementation of independent nurse prescribers is to make better use of the nurses' skills as well as making it easier for patients to get access to the medicines they need.

The area associated with nurse prescribing is constantly changing and will continue to do so in the future. Specific programmes of study are provided by institutions of higher education that prepare nurses to take on the role of independent prescriber. These programmes of study must be approved by the NMC as well as the Royal Pharmaceutical Society of Great Britain.

> **Activity 2.21 Reflection**
>
> Take some time when in clinical practice to reflect on the issue of medicines management; choose an activity that you can use to reflect upon. In the box below, write what happened, how you felt, and what you would do differently (if anything) next time you are involved in the management of medications.
>
> **What happened?**
>
> **How did it make you feel?**
>
> **What would you do differently (if anything) next time?**

Chapter summary

Safe and effective nursing care involves the safe and effective administration of medicines and the student nurse needs to develop the skills, knowledge and attitude required to do this in order to administer medicines legally and safely when he/she qualifies as a registered nurse. During nurse education, the student can administer medicines but this must only be carried out under the direct supervision of a registered nurse or registered midwife.

The student nurse must understand the importance of administering medicines in a safe and competent manner, developing and building on skills and knowledge, understanding the various routes of administration and the pharmacokinetics underpinning medicine management. The nurse has a responsibility for assessing, planning, implementing and evaluating care in relation to medicines management. The administration of medicines also provides the nurse with the opportunity to engage with the patient providing education about drug regimens.

No medication can be given to a patient without a prescription (or a direction to supply) from a licensed practitioner; to do otherwise would be illegal. There are many statutory requirements that govern and inform safe drug administration including domestic UK law and European directives.

The NMC provide much guidance relating to the administration of medicines and medicine management. This guidance can help the nurse ensure that he/she is practicing within the realms of the NMC Code (2008b) and upholding its central tenet to act in the patient's best interests in order to do no harm.

Answers to Activities

Activity 2.1 Key terms

Using a nursing or medical dictionary or any other resource you think may help you; begin this chapter by finding out the meaning of the words below. You might want to make use of the human resources around you, for example registered nurses, pharmacist or doctor. There are blank spaces provided for you to enter your responses.

Term	Definition
Allergy	Disorder of the immune system
Anaphylaxis	A severe allergic reaction
Balm	A topical medical preparation
Buccal	Relating to the cheeks or mouth cavity
Contraindication	A reason that makes it inadvisable to prescribe a particular drug
Epidural	An injection into the epidural space of the spine
Half-life	The time required for something to fall to half of its initial value
Hypodermic	Related to or below the epidermis
Hypodermoclysis	Subcutaneous injection of a fluid, i.e. saline
Intradermal	Within or between the layers of the skin
Transdermal patch	A medicated adhesive that is placed on the skin to deliver a time released dose of medication through the skin and into the blood stream
Intramuscular	Within the substance of a muscle
Intraocular	Within the eye (eye ball)
Intraosseous	Within a bone
Intravenous	Within a vein
Lotion	A liquid for external application to the body
Ointment	A highly viscous or semisolid preparation for external application
Pessary	A medicated vaginal suppository
Subcutaneous	Beneath the skin
Sublingual	Below or beneath the tongue
Suppository	A medicated plug of medication for insertion into a body cavity, i.e. the rectum

Activity 2.1 (*Continued*)

Intra-aural	Within the ear
Intra-vesicular	Within the bladder
Suspension	Finely divided, undissolved particles in a liquid medium, must also be shaken prior to administration
Solution	A drug dissolved in another solution, a liquid preparation
Cream	A spreadable substance similar to ointment but not as thick
Capsule	Powder or gel form of an active drug
Tablet	A solid dosage form containing a medicine
Enema	A solution introduced into the rectum
Syrup	A medication combined in a water and sugar solution
Elixir	A hydro-alcoholic liquid containing a medicinal agent, sweeteners and flavours
Nebuliser	A devise creating an aerosol usually with a medicinal agent added
Inhaler	An apparatus for administering a vapour or volatilised medicinal agent

Activities 2.2, 2.3 and 2.4 are personal to you.

Activity 2.5

Make a list of those people who you think are authorised under the Misuse of Drugs Regulations 2001 to supply and/or possess controlled drugs while acting in their professional capacities.

Some of those people who are authorised under the Misuse of Drugs Regulations 2001 to supply and/or possess controlled drugs while acting in their professional capacities are:

- Practitioner pharmacist
- Doctor
- Public analyst
- Nurse
- Dentist
- Owner of a nursing home
- Midwife
- Vet
- Person in charge of a hospital

Go to this website to find out more about the Misuse of Drugs Regulations 2001: http://www.opsi.gov.uk/si/si2001/20013998.htm

Activity 2.6

Below is a list of drugs that fall under the ABC classificatory system. See if you can arrange them in their classificatory order, where class A drugs are said to cause most risk and carry heavier penalties for possession and supply.

Ecstasy	Gamma-hydroxybutyrate (GHB)	Methylphenidate (Ritalin)
Methyl amphetamine	Anabolic steroids	Barbiturate
Codeine	Crack cocaine	Magic mushrooms
LSD	Amphetamines	Temazepam
Barbiturates	Cocaine	Cannabis
Heroin	Amphetamines (for injection)	Diazepam

Ketamine

The classification of a selection of controlled drugs along with the maximum penalties associated with illegal possession and supply is provided in Table 2.5.

Table 2.5   A section of controlled drugs, their classifications and the maximum penalties associated with their possession and supply
(*Source:* Adapted from House of Commons, 2006).

Class	Drugs	Maximum penalties
A	Heroin LSD Ecstasy Amphetamines (for injection) Cocaine Crack cocaine Magic mushrooms	For possession: 7 years imprisonment and/or fine For supply: life imprisonment and/or fine
B	Amphetamines Methyl amphetamines Barbiturates Codeine	For possession: 5 years imprisonment and/or fine For supply: 14 years imprisonment and/or a fine
C	Cannabis Temazepam Anabolic steroids Diazepam Ketamine Methylphenidate (Ritalin) Gamma-hydroxybutyrate (GHB)	For possession: 2 years imprisonment and/or fine For supply: 14 years imprisonment and/or fine

Activity 2.7

Example: SI units

1. Convert 300 mg into grams	Answer: 300 mg = 0.3 g
2. Convert 750 micrograms into mg	Answer: 750 mcg = 0.75 mg

Here are some more:

1. Convert 400 mg into grams	Answer: 0.4 g
2. Convert 850 micrograms into mg	Answer: 0.85 mg
3. Convert 250 mg to g	Answer: 0.25 g
4. Convert 0.5 g to mg	Answer: 500 mg
5. Convert 250 mcg to mg	Answer: 0.25 mg
6. Convert 50 mL to litres	Answer: 0.05 L
7. Convert 0.125 g to mg	Answer: 125 mg

Activity 2.8 Total fluid balance

Getwell Hospital
Fluid Balance Chart

Name..

Ward...

Hospital number..

DoB...

Time	Input (in mL)		Output (in mL)		
	Intravenous	Oral/other	Urine	Other	Comments
0000	2.60	NBM	20		
0100	2.65		10	1.20	Nasogastric
0200	2.75		10		
0300	3.84		8.2		
0400	8.70		2.6		
0500	6.00		8.0	1.80	Nasogastric
0600	6.00		12.2		
0700	9.90		10.2		
0800	3.65		10		
0900	7.75		14	1.10	Nasogastric
1000	12.00		13		
1100	12.75		14.7		
1200	20.00		12.4		
1300	21.20		20	1.20	Nasogastric
1400	22.00		32		

(continued)

Activity 2.8 (*Continued*)

Time	Input (in mL)		Output (in mL)		
	Intravenous	Oral/other	Urine	Other	Comments
1500	75.00		36		
1600	75.00		26		
1700	15.00		28	1.75	Nasogastric
1800	0.75		23		
1900	0.75		22		
2000	1.75		18		
2100	10.75		12.8	1.80	Nasogastric
2200	20.75		14.6		
2300	21.75		12.4		
Total	363.29	Nil	390.1	8.85	

Urine output is 26.81 mL more that input.

Activity 2.9 is self-explanatory.

Activity 2.10

1. **If a patient requires 20 mg and each tablet is 5 mg, how many tablets are required?**
   Answer: 4
2. **A patient is prescribed 1.5 g of Flucloxacillin; stock available is 750 mg capsules. How many capsules does the patient require?**
   Answer: 2
3. **A patient is prescribed 120 mg of Frusemide, the tablets available are 40 mg. How many tablets are required?**
   Answer: 3
4. **A 50 mg dose is prescribed; tablets are 12.5 mg each. How many tablets will you give?**
   Answer: 4
5. **A 625 mg dose is prescribed; tablets are 1.25 g each. How many tablets will you give?**
   Answer: 1/2
6. **A 150 mg dose is prescribed; tablets are 50 mg each. How many tablets will you give?**
   Answer: 3
7. **A 75 mg dose is prescribed; tablets are 25 mg each. How many would you give?**
   Answer: 3
8. **A 25 mg dose is prescribed; tablets are 12.5 mg each. How many would you give?**
   Answer: 2
9. **A 1 mg dose is prescribed; tablets are 500 micrograms. How many tablets will you give?**
   Answer: 2
10. **Three tablets each contain 250 mg. What is the total dose in milligrams?**
    Answer: 750 mg

Activity 2.11

There are no answers to this activity as you have been asked to use the British National Formulary to learn how to use that publication and also to learn about the various medicines, the comments here are prompts

Drug	Generic and/or propriety name	Adult dose	Route(s) of administration	Contra-indications	Side effects	Category
Paracetamol	What name(s) are used for paracetamol–there are many	Look at the various ranges of dose	There are number of routes of administration	These contraindications may surprise you	There are several side effects listed for this commonly used medicine	Choose POM, P, GSL, Controlled Drug
Diamorphine	This drug has several propriety names	The adult dose will vary based on several factors	There are several routes of administration. The fastest acting route is the intravenous route	You need to be aware of these in order to practice safely	Side effects associated with medicine are numerous	Choose POM, P, GSL, Controlled Drug
Diazepam	There is one commonly used propriety name for this medicine	There are standard doses, but these must take account of the individual's specific needs	There is a usual route of administration, but there are also other routes depending on the need for the drug	Contraindications vary with this medicine	As with most drugs diazepam has a number of different side effects	Choose POM, P, GSL, Controlled Drug
Buscopan	What are the various names used for this medicine	Doses are matched to patient need and other important factors	The preferred route of administration for this medicine may interest you	It is important to be aware of these in order to practice safely	Some side effects may be negated by choosing an alternative route of administration	Choose POM, P, GSL, Controlled Drug

Activity 2.12

Can you think of any other oral medications?
You may have considered:

- Pills
- Lozenges
- Capsules
- Solution
- Elixir

Activity 2.13

When administering oral medications, what equipment is required?
When administering oral medications, the equipment that is required is:

- Prescription chart
- Medication
- Medicine pot with measured graduations
- Water
- Oral syringe
- Measuring spoon with measured graduations
- Drug formulary, for example the BNF

Activity 2.14

Try these oral drug calculations:

1. Patient requires analgesia. He can have Paracetamol Elixir 500 mg. The elixir contains 250 mg in 10 mL. How many millilitres will he require?
   Answer: 20 mL
2. If a patient required 100 mg and each bottle contains 250 mg in 5 mL, how much do you give?
   Answer: 2 mL
3. Sodium valporate oral solution is supplied as 200 mg/5 mL. The patient requires 300 mg. How many millilitres does the patient require?
   Answer: 7.5 mL
4. If a patient required 250 mg and each bottle contains 125 mg in 5 mL, how much do you give?
   Answer: 10 mL
5. Linctus is available as 25 mg in 5 mL and we need to give the patient 75 mg. What volume will be given?
   Answer: 15 mL

Activity 2.15

Some advantages and disadvantages of intravenous medication:

Advantages	Disadvantages
• Provides high blood levels of the drug • Can be used when the person is unable to swallow • The medication can be absorbed directly into the blood stream as opposed to via the gastrointestinal tract when absorption through this route is impossible • The drug is rapidly absorbed • Can be less traumatic for the patient who requires a number of injections, for example, via the intramuscular route	• Contamination on insertion and whilst the intravenous device is *in situ* • The drug is rapidly absorbed • Extravasation and phlebitis • Air embolism • Fluid overload • Can restrict mobility, thus rendering the patient dependent • Requires specific nursing care whilst infusion device or infusion is in progress • Anaphylaxis

Activity 2.16

Look at these diagrams (see Figure 2.3) and see where the muscles described above are situated?

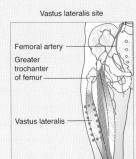

Vastus lateralis site

Femoral artery
Greater trochanter of femur
Vastus lateralis

Dorsogluteal site

Posterior superior iliac spine
Gluteus medius
Gluteus minimus
Gluteus maximus
Greater trochanter of femur
Sciatic nerve

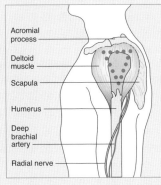

Deltoid site

Acromial process
Deltoid muscle
Scapula
Humerus
Deep brachial artery
Radial nerve

Activity 2.17

Drug calculations for injections

1. A client is ordered 45 mg of Loxapine by intramuscular injection. A 50 mg dose in 1 mL of liquid for IM Injection is available. How many millilitres will you administer?
   Answer: 0.9 mL
2. A client is ordered Pethidine 35 mg IM as a pre-medication. Stock ampoules contain 50 mg per mL. What volume must be withdrawn for injection?
   Answer: 0.7 mL
3. A client is ordered 100 mg by intramuscular injection. A 50 mg dose in 1 mL of liquid for IM Injection is available. How many millilitres will you administer?
   Answer: 2 mL
4. A client is ordered 25 mg by intramuscular injection. A 50 mg dose in 1 mL of liquid for IM Injection is available. How many millilitres will you administer?
   Answer: 0.5 mL
5. A client is ordered 300 mg by intramuscular injection. A 100 mg dose in 1 mL of liquid for IM Injection is available. How many millilitres will you administer?
   Answer: 3 mL

Activity 2.18

What factors would you consider when giving a subcutaneous injection?
Factors to consider when giving a subcutaneous injection:

- Wash your hands prior to giving the injection.
- Provide the patient with dignity by ensuring that doors are closed, curtains drawn.
- Explain the procedure to the patient.
- Ensure that there is sufficient lighting and the height of the bed has been adjusted to ensure that you are ergonomically safe.
- Position the patient for the injection, exposing minimal anatomy.
- Put gloves on.
- Clean the site of injection with an alcohol wipe if this is policy using a circular action. There are some types of subcutaneous injection that do not require skin cleansing.
- Remove the needle guard (sheath) ensuring that the needle only touches the inside of the guard.
- Stretch the skin taut, with the other hand over the injection site.
- Holding the syringe like a dart, insert the needle into the skin quickly at the correct angle; usually for subcutaneous injection, this is a 90° angle or 45° if the patient is very thin in order to ensure that the needle does not pierce the muscle.
- Inject the medication by pushing the plunger slowly into the barrel with even pressure.
- Steady the patient's tissue that is immediately adjacent to the puncture site with your other hand and quickly remove the needle.
- If it is policy, gently massage the injection site with an alcohol wipe.
- Lower the bed if it has been elevated and leave the patient comfortable.
- Never resheath or replace the needle guard, dispose of the used needle and syringe into the nearest sharps box in accordance with policy.
- Complete all necessary documentation.

Activity 2.19

What are creams, ointments, lotions, liniments and powders required for?

Creams
Lotions
Ointments
Liniments
Powders (talc)

These types of medicine are often required to treat skin conditions and are called topical medications; they are administered externally onto the body as opposed to being ingested or injected. Medicines applied to the nose and ear are also topical medicines. Topical medicines should not be applied near the eyes or mouth; they can cause stinging and are not to be taken orally. Different preparations have different modes of action. Lotions protect, soften, soothe and can provide relief from itching. Ointments are oil based and body heat causes them to melt after they have been applied; often medications that are used to fight infection or soothe inflamed tissue. Liniments provide relief to tight aching muscles and are applied by rubbing.

Most skin medications are provided for use in tubes; one tube one patient use can help to prevent cross infection. Some skin medications must be sterile for use, and if this is the case after application, the remaining medication left in the tube must be discarded. The six Rs outlined in Table 2.4 apply to the administration of topical medications as well, ensuring that the strength of the medicine is the correct strength.

Gloves should be used when applying creams, ointments and lotions and they should be applied sparingly. The medication must be applied in thin even layers unless the prescription dictates otherwise; a thick coating can prevent air that is necessary for healing from reaching the wound. The area to be treated should be cleansed prior to the application of the medicine with warm water or a gentle mild soap. When applying the medication, care should be taken not to increase discomfort by using undue pressure or rubbing the areas that are inflamed or painful.

Activity 2.20

There are several reasons why a person may need to have ophthalmic medications. List below what you think these may be.
You may have considered:

- To treat eye disease
- To soothe tissue
- To dilate or constrict the pupil
- To provide anaesthetic

Activity 2.21 Reflection

Take some time when in clinical practice to reflect on the issue of medicines management; choose an activity that you can use to reflect upon. In the box below, write what happened, how you felt, and what you would do differently (if anything) next time you are involved in the management of medications.

What happened?

● Describe the scenario briefly relating to your learning need.

How did it make you feel?

● Did you feel good or bad about it?
● What was good or bad about the situation?
● Did you have adequate underpinning knowledge to carry out the care?
● If you had previous experience of similar situation, was it useful this time?

What would you do differently (if anything) next time?

● Has this personal experience prepared you to do further reading and gained more practice under supervision?

This is only a guide. Please address the sub-headings to meet your own learning needs.

References

Ahmed, I. and Majeed, A. (2007) The safe and responsible disposal of unused controlled drugs. *British Journal of Nursing* **16** (21), 1381–1322.

Department of Health (2004a) *Building a Safer NHS for Patients: Improving Medication Safety* (London: DH).

Department of Health (2004b) *Building a Safer NHS for Patients: Improving Medication Safety. A Report by the Chief Pharmaceutical Officer* (London: DH).

Department of Health (2006a) *Safer Management of Controlled Drugs: Changes to Record Keeping Requirements (Final Guidance)* (London: DH).

Department of Health (2006b) *Medicine Matters: A guide to the Mechanism for the Prescribing, Supply and Administration of Medicines* (London: DH).

Ellis, J.R. and Bentz, P.M. (2007) *Modules for Basic Nursing Skills*, 7th edn (Philadelphia: Lippincott).

Gray, J. and Jackson, C. (2004) The development of an online quiz for drug calculations. *Nursing Times* **100** (4), 40–41.

Griffith, R., Griffith, H. and Jordan, S. (2003) Administration of medicines: Part 1. *Nursing Standard* **18** (2), 47–53.

House of Commons (2006) *Science and Technology — Fifth Report* (London: House of Commons).

Hutton, M. (2005) *Calculation Skills: Paediatric Dosages* (London: RCN Publishing Company).

Modernisation Agency (2005) *Medicine Matters: A Guide to Current Mechanisms for the Prescribing, Supply and Administration of Medicines* (London: Modernisation Agency).

Nursing and Midwifery Council (2002) *An NMC for Students for Nursing and Midwifery* (London: NMC).

Nursing and Midwifery Council (2005) *Standards of Proficiency for Nurse and Midwife Prescribers* (London: NMC).

Nursing and Midwifery Council (2006) *Covert Administration of Medicines: Advice Sheet* (London: NMC).

Nursing and Midwifery Council (2008a) *Standards for Medicines Management* (London: NMC).

Nursing and Midwifery Council (2008b) *The Code: Standards of Conduct, Performance and Ethics for Nurses and Midwives* (London: NMC).

Quinn, C. (2000) Infusion devices: risks, functions and management. *Nursing Standard* **14** (26), 35–41.

Trim, J. (2004) Clinical skills; a practical guide to working out drug calculations. *British Journal of Nursing* **13** (10), 602–606.

Weeks, K.W., Lyne, P. and Torrance, C. (2000) Written drug dosage errors made by students: the threat to clinical effectiveness and the need for a new approach. *Clinical Effectiveness in Nursing* **4**, 20–29.

Woodrow, P. (1998) Numeracy skills. *Nursing Standard* **10** (6), 26–30.

Wright, K. (2004) An investigation to find strategies to improve student nurses' maths skills. *British Journal of Nursing* **13** (21), 1280–1284.

Useful websites

Nursing and Midwifery Council: www.nmc-uk.org

Department of Health (England): www.dh.gov.uk

The Scottish Executive: www.scotland.gov.uk

The Welsh Assembly: www.wales.gov.uk

Department of Health and Social Services and Patient Safety of Northern Ireland: www.dhsspsni.gov.uk

Community and District Nurses Association: www.cdna-online.org.uk

Community Practitioners and Health Visitors Association: www.amicus-cphv.org

Royal College of Nursing: www.rcn.org.uk

Royal Pharmaceutical Society of Great Britain: www.rpsgb.org.uk

Royal Pharmaceutical Society of Northern Ireland: www.dotphramacy.com.psni

Scottish Pharmaceutical General Council: www.rspgc.org.uk/scotland

Principles of monitoring and assessment

HELEN BARNETT

> ## Aims
>
> The aim of this chapter is to introduce you to the key principles of monitoring and assessment. It will also provide you with an overview of the planning, implementing and evaluating of vital signs.

> ## Learning objectives
>
> On completion of this chapter, you will learn:
> - The principles of assessing, planning, implementing and evaluating care
> - How to set appropriate goals as part of the care planning process
> - The normal values when assessing vital signs
> - How to recognise deviations from the norm when assessing vital signs
> - The factors affecting vital signs
> - The principles of documentation as part of assessment and monitoring

---

Introduction

Monitoring and assessment are essential parts of nursing practice and underpin the care we deliver in any setting. Assessment of individuals allows us to gather information about the person. Monitoring allows nurses to establish if a person's well-being or situation is improving, static or worsening. The assessment and monitoring of people enables nurses to identify the person's

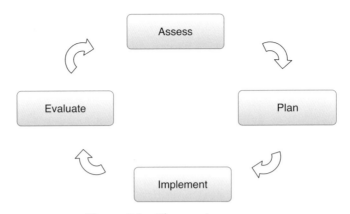

Figure 3.1   The nursing process

individual needs and to plan and implement care which is tailored to meet these needs. This chapter will examine these processes and enable you to revise your knowledge of these stages which constitute the nursing process.

The assessment and monitoring of vital signs is an important aspect of nursing care which provides essential physiological data and therefore information about a person's condition. Physiological observations are important in recognising if a person's condition is static, deteriorating or indeed improving (Kisiel and Perkins, 2006). Vital signs usually encompass respiratory rate, temperature, pulse and blood pressure. This chapter will address these in further detail and give you an opportunity to revise your knowledge of each. You will also be given opportunities to reflect on your own practice in relation to vital signs. However, it is important to recognise that assessment of any person will involve the collection of a much wider array of information. Other physiological data may include urine output, oxygen saturations, peak flow readings and neurological assessment. In addition, the assessment process is likely to gather information relating to the person's physical, social, psychological and spiritual well-being. This chapter will consider the assessment process in its broadest sense.

Assessment is only the initial stage of the nursing process which encompasses the four stages identified in Figure 3.1.

The nursing process underpins everyday nursing practice and ensures that care delivery is systematically organised to meet a person's individual needs. It is a dynamic and ongoing process and can therefore be presented in a cyclical manner (Figure 3.1). In some cases, the nursing process may incorporate five phases with the addition of a nursing diagnosis following assessment. A nursing diagnosis involves the identification of actual or potential needs based on the information collated within the assessment. It is important to recognise that diagnosis is not unique to the medical profession. Nurses are able to use their knowledge, skills and experience to identify health problems upon which care should be planned and implemented.

In summary, the nursing process provides a framework to underpin nursing practice. Adopting a systematic approach to care is essential in ensuring that people receive the highest quality care that is responsive to their individual needs and continuously evaluated and amended as required.

Assessment of vital signs

Key terms

It is important to understand the medical terminology relating to vital signs.

Activity 3.1 Key terms

Use your nursing dictionary to look up the following terms and provide a complete definition of each term.

Term	Definition
Tachypnoeic	
Bradypnoeic	
Apnoeic	
Tachycardic	
Bradycardic	
Hypertensive	
Hypotensive	
Pyrexial	
Apyrexial	
Hyperthermic	
Hypothermic	

The assessment of vital signs is an important skill which will enable the collection of important physiological data. Vital signs are key measurements that may be influenced by physical, emotional and environmental factors. Overall, they provide an indication of the state of core physical functions, namely respiratory rate, temperature, pulse and blood pressure. It is important that such measurements are taken and recorded with complete accuracy as the care that is implemented may produce changes in vital signs. For example, if you record that a person's blood pressure is elevated, medication may be prescribed to reduce this. This has to be monitored closely to ensure that blood pressure does not fall to an unsafe level. Likewise, McAlister and Straus (2001) highlight that if blood pressure is consistently underestimated, many people with hypertension (elevated blood pressure) could be denied potentially life-saving treatment. There are numerous ways to record vital signs. Spend a few moments thinking about the vital signs you have measured in practice and the challenges that you faced.

Activity 3.2

Make a note of some of your thoughts. For example, you may have tried to record a person's vital signs but felt very anxious about explaining your findings to the person.

Respiratory rate

The primary function of breathing is to supply the body with oxygen and to remove carbon dioxide. Any change in a person's ability to breathe normally may affect his or her ability to perform this vital function. One respiration consists of both an inspiration and expiration. An altered respiratory rate is often deemed to be a most useful and early sign of a change in a person's condition. This is because the respiratory system is most sensitive to changes in oxygen and carbon dioxide and will be altered as an immediate compensatory mechanism. Respiratory rate, therefore, gives a baseline of ventilatory function and an early indication of deterioration (Kenward, 2001; Butler-Williams, 2005). However, there is significant evidence that respiratory rate is often poorly documented in a person's observations (Chellel *et al.*, 2002, Hodgetts *et al.*, 2002). In addition to respiratory rate, it may be necessary to conduct a full respiratory assessment including breathing pattern, depth, breath sounds and oxygen saturations. A more detailed explanation of respiratory care is provided in Chapter 4.

Activity 3.3

Write down some of the key considerations when assessing a person's respiratory rate.

Top tip

To avoid the patient being aware that you are measuring his or her respiratory rate, try measuring it directly after you have taken the radial pulse whilst still holding the patient's wrist.

Temperature

Body temperature is regulated by the hypothalamus in the brain. It is the balance between the heat produced and the heat lost from the body. The body requires a stable core temperature to maintain cell metabolic activity (Trim, 2005). There are two kinds of body temperature: core

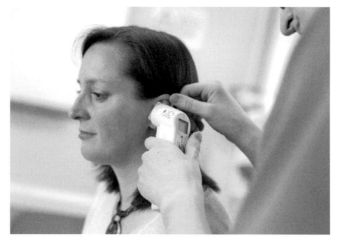

Figure 3.2   Taking a temperature from the ear

temperature and surface temperature (Kozier *et al.*, 2008). Most often in clinical practice you will measure the surface temperature which is the temperature of the skin, subcutaneous tissue and fat. It is also possible to measure core temperature of the deep tissues of the body such as the abdominal cavity and pelvic cavity (Kozier *et al.*, 2008). Unlike surface temperature (which will alter in response to the environment), core temperature is likely to remain relatively constant. It is most useful in monitoring critically ill patients, for whom it may be necessary to use an invasive device to measure temperature. You may have seen surface body temperature assessed using a number of different recording sites including oral, rectal, axillary (armpit) and tympanic membrane (ear) (see Figure 3.2). The choice of site depends on the person whom you are assessing.

Activity 3.4

Identify some of the advantages and disadvantages of using these four recording sites.

	Advantages	Disadvantages
Oral		

(continued)

Activity 3.4 (*Continued*)

	Advantages	Disadvantages
Rectal		
Axillary		
Tympanic membrane		

You may have seen a variety of devices used to measure body temperature.

Mercury-filled thermometers

In some areas you may still see mercury-filled glass thermometers. These are now less common, as it is recognised that both the glass and mercury present a potential hazard.

Electronic thermometers

Electronic thermometers have replaced mercury-filled devices in many areas. These often have a probe that can be used for oral, axilla or rectal readings. A disposable cover is often used for each use, or the probes are colour-coded to differentiate the site it is to be used for. Regardless of the site selected, the accuracy of the reading is dependent on correct probe placement and the cleanliness of the equipment (Carroll, 2000).

Disposable thermometers

There are a number of disposable thermometers available, which are particularly useful in community and home settings. The most common types are the chemical dot thermometer and liquid crystal heat-sensitive synthetic strip.

Infrared thermometers

The most common type of infrared thermometer is used to measure temperature within the ear canal. They detect infrared energy that is emitted from the tympanic membrane at the end of the ear and surrounding tissues (Jamieson *et al.*, 2007). Normally a disposable cover is placed over the probe before insertion into the ear canal.

Pulse

A pulse is a rhythmic expansion and recoil of the elastic arteries caused by the ejection of blood from the left ventricle (Jamieson *et al.*, 2007). This ejected blood passes through the aorta and into the body's general circulation. When assessing the pulse, it is important to take note of the rate, rhythm and strength of the pulsation. Under normal circumstances, the peripheral pulse rate you are measuring will directly correspond with the patient's heart rate (apical rate). A discrepancy between the two may indicate vascular disease and will require further investigation. When noting the rhythm of the pulse, it is important to consider whether the pulse you are feeling is regular throughout the duration of your assessment. If a pulse rate is irregular, the patient is said to have an arrhythmia or dysrhythmia which could be a sign of an underlying condition. It is therefore important not to rely on electronic devices such as pulse oximeters (which also give an indication of heart rate) as these will not provide information about the rhythm and strength of the heart rate. When assessing the strength of the pulse, it is important to think about whether the pulse you are feeling is weak, thready or bounding. If you detect any abnormalities in the assessment of the pulse, it will be necessary to seek medical advice. It may then be appropriate to complete a more detailed cardiac assessment to include cardiac monitoring or a 12 lead electrocardiogram. There are numerous pulse points within the body. These are sites where a large artery lies close to the skin and the pulse can be palpated.

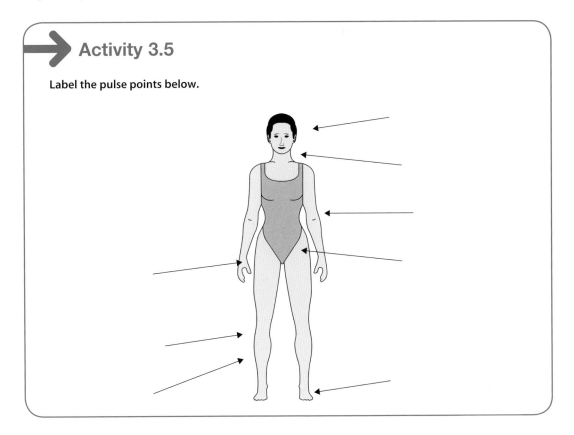

→ Activity 3.5

Label the pulse points below.

Now spend a few moments reflecting on your clinical practice.

> ### ➤ Activity 3.6
>
> **Reflect on your practice and record the sites you have used to measure a person's pulse and the reasons why this might have been.**

Often the most common pulse point used in clinical practice is the radial pulse (which is one of the peripheral pulses). This is because it is easily accessible. However, there may have been occasions when you have used another pulse site. For example, in a person who is rapidly deteriorating, it is often preferable to use the carotid pulse. This is because the heart will continue to supply blood to the brain for as long as possible whilst peripheral pulses may have weakened and be less easy to palpate. Likewise in a baby or young child, you may take the apex pulse (a central pulse) using a stethoscope over the heart, as the peripheral pulses are often difficult to palpate.

> ### ➤ Activity 3.7
>
> **Reflect on taking a person's radial pulse and the considerations you would make.**

Blood pressure

Blood pressure is the pressure exerted by the blood on the walls of a blood vessel (Hogston and Marjoram, 2007). Blood pressure is essential in driving the blood around the body and allowing the delivery of oxygen to body tissues. Blood pressure is measured for a variety of reasons including routine checks, during hospital admission or outpatient attendance, as part of chronic disease management such as cardiovascular disease or diabetes, during pregnancy and in the monitoring of hypertension (Hinckley and Walker, 2005).

Activity 3.8

Label the diagram of the heart.

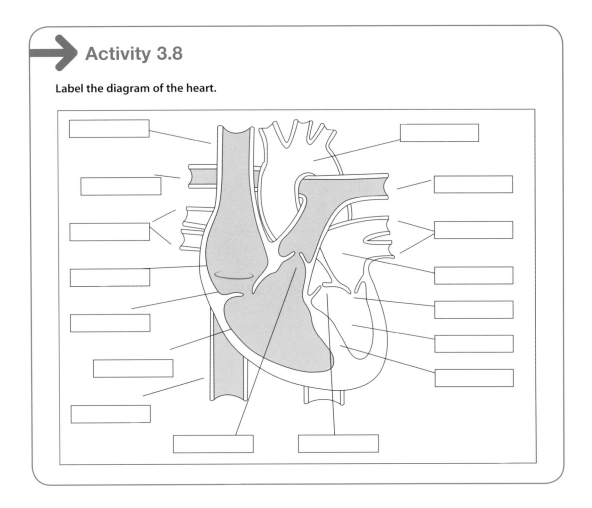

In most cases, arterial blood pressure is recorded and two readings are taken: the systolic and diastolic blood pressure.

Activity 3.9

Define these two terms and identify the related physiology.

	Definition
Systolic	
Diastolic	

There are several methods used to assess a person's blood pressure, which include both direct and indirect monitoring.

Manual reading (using a sphygmomanometer)

The use of a sphygmomanometer is generally an accurate method by which to monitor blood pressure indirectly. However, these devices may be less common in your clinical area. Often they have been replaced with automated devices. One of the reasons for this is that some manual devices with a sphygmomanometer contain mercury which is a highly toxic material. Once in the environment, mercury accumulates in food chains and is dangerous as a vapour (Simpson, 2006). In some settings, the mercury devices have been replaced by aneroid devices which also require you to listen for changes in blood flow as the cuff is released.

It is important that you develop competency in this form of blood pressure assessment as you may need to use it in settings such as the community, or if the automated equipment is faulty.

Automated devices

These electronic devices are used to measure blood pressure indirectly, and are now commonly used in clinical areas (see Figure 3.3) and people's homes. It is important that they are used in accordance with manufacturer's guidelines and that the cuff is positioned accurately. There are occasions when this method may be unsuitable. One such example is if the pulse is weak and thready, as this may not be detected by an automated device.

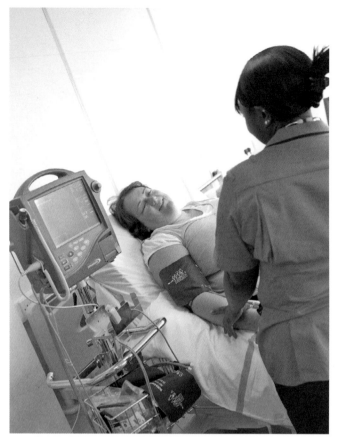

Figure 3.3   Taking an electronic blood pressure

Continuous invasive monitoring

These direct methods of monitoring blood pressure involve the insertion of a cannula into an artery and the use of a pressure transducing unit. Direct blood pressure monitoring is most accurate, but requires continuous observation and clinical expertise on behalf of the nurse. These methods are reserved for use in specialist areas (such as theatres or intensive care units) in the care of critically ill people and those requiring more advanced monitoring.

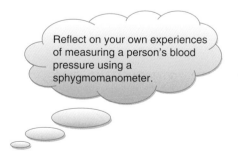

Reflect on your own experiences of measuring a person's blood pressure using a sphygmomanometer.

Activity 3.10

Label the equipment shown in the figure below. Try to list the purpose of each part of the equipment.

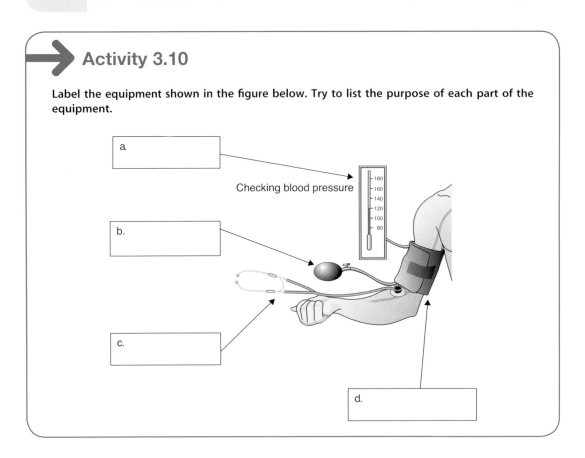

a.

Checking blood pressure

b.

c.

d.

Activity 3.11

Make a list of the key considerations whilst taking a blood pressure.

Regardless of the methods used, it is vital that blood pressure is measured and recorded accurately. This is to ensure that the results give an accurate indication of the patient's physiological state (Castledine, 2006). Errors in blood pressure measurement are often the result of poor technique or faulty equipment (Wallymahmed, 2008). One consideration you may have noted above is the position of the patient. A study by Eşer *et al.* (2006) concluded that body position affected the accuracy of blood pressure measurement in healthy young adults, and recommended that blood pressure should be taken in a sitting position with the arm supported at the right atrial level. Whilst the use of automated devices is now widespread, it is important to recognise the limitations. For example, these devices are not suitable for patients with an irregular heart rate (O'Brien *et al.*, 2003). Nurses should, therefore, remain skilled in using manual devices, and have a choice of devices at their disposal (Cork, 2007). It may be useful to refer to the British Hypertension Society (BHS) and the Medicines and Healthcare products Regulatory Agency (MHRA) for detailed guidance on accurate blood pressure measurement.

Early warning scores (EWS)

It is now recognised that when a person's condition deteriorates, he or she displays common signs that represent failing respiratory, cardiovascular and neurological systems (Resuscitation Council UK, 2005). Therefore, the accurate assessment of vital signs is essential in ensuring that people at risk of becoming critically ill are recognised at the earliest opportunity, and that appropriate care is planned and implemented. In recent years, early warning scores (EWS) or 'calling-criteria' have been adopted by many hospitals to assist in the early detection of critical illness (McArthur-Rouse, 2001). EWS systems require you to allocate a score to each vital sign according to its deviation from the norm. These scores allow healthcare professionals to recognise when a person's condition is deteriorating and further intervention is required. For example, the EWS system may require you to contact the critical care outreach team for further support.

Principles of assessment of care

Assessment of the person is the first stage of the nursing process and involves the collection of information to guide the planning of care. Whilst it is identified as the first stage of the nursing process, it is important to remember that assessment is ongoing as we continually collect information about the patient, and assess responses to the care we implement. Information may relate to a person's physical, psychological, social, emotional and spiritual well-being. A thorough assessment is vital in ensuring that appropriate care is planned which meets an individual's needs. For example, in your *physical* assessment of a person you may establish that he or she has longstanding pain in his or her left hip and that the medical plan of care is to perform joint replacement surgery. You may plan to aim for discharge after 3 days. However, your assessment of the *social* aspects of the person's life may have revealed that he or she lives in a flat on the sixth floor and currently has no access to a lift. This aspect of the assessment will have significant implications for the subsequent care that is planned and implemented related to rehabilitation and discharge planning. Your assessment will also include both objective and subjective information. In this case, an example of objective information would be the patient's vital signs. Subjective data may include the patient reporting 'I feel unwell' or 'I feel miserable'. Both of these types of information are vital in planning holistic care for the patient.

The information you collect may require you to use a range of methods and some specific assessment tools. An assessment tool provides a structured approach to collecting information about a specific aspect of a patient's care. One example is the use of a scale to assess the risk of pressure ulcer development such as that by Waterlow (2005). This tool allows you to assess the level of risk the patient has of developing a pressure ulcer by identifying the contributing factors. Care can then be planned based on the severity of the risk. Objective risk assessment measurement scales have been recommended by the UK Department of Health (2003) as part of *Essence of Care*.

Activity 3.12

Write down some examples of assessment tools that you have seen used in practice.

Your assessment of any person is likely to require you to use a range of skills to enable you to gather sensitive and accurate information about the person.

Activity 3.13

Think about the assessments you have seen in practice and list some of the skills that you used.

You may have identified communication skills in your list above. Communication skills are extremely important when assessing a person. Consider the responses you may receive when asking a person the following questions:

1. Do you find it alright to catch the bus to the day centre each day?
2. How do you feel about your journey to the day centre each day?

The first question is a closed question and is likely to elicit a 'yes' or 'no' answer. You will then have limited information upon which to plan care with the person. However, the second question is an open question and invites the person to tell you anything related to his or her journey. Whilst he or she may have responded 'yes' to the first question, the use of an open question may enable you to understand much more about the journey including duration, cost, ease of use, convenience and so on. This provides a more meaningful and insightful assessment of that aspect of a person's life.

Activity 3.14

Write an example of a closed and open question. Think about the types of response do you think each would elicit.

Closed question

Open question

Many healthcare professionals are likely to be involved in the assessment of a person. In recent years, there has been a move towards a single assessment process (SAP) to avoid duplication of assessment. This was introduced as part of the National Service Framework for Older People (Department of Health, 2001). SAP aims to ensure that individuals are placed at the heart of the assessment process and that this is timely and in proportion to individuals' needs.

Principles of planning of care

The second phase of the nursing process is the planning of care. This should be based on the assessment of the person you have undertaken and should aim to meet the needs of that person. The planning of care involves the setting of achievable goals and planning how they can best be achieved (Kenworthy *et al.*, 2002). In some circumstances, it may be necessary to follow recognised national guidelines when planning a patient's care. For example, the National Institute for Health and Clinical Excellence (NICE) has produced a number of guidelines relating to certain conditions. If your initial assessment has revealed that the patient has sustained a head injury, for example, it will be necessary to adhere to the NICE guidelines when planning the frequency of vital sign measurements and other nursing activities. Whenever possible, it is important to involve the person in the planning of his or her own care and to ensure that he or she understands the plan that is formulated. This is often referred to as person-centred goal setting. People have a right, and often a desire, to be involved in their own care. An awareness of their goals will enable them to be more actively involved in their care and may lead them to be more motivated. This may potentially enhance and accelerate their recovery.

In many cases, you are likely to have identified a number of needs in your initial assessment. This then requires these needs to be prioritised. Prioritisation means opting for one thing and discarding or postponing another (Werntoft *et al.*, 2005). In nursing, this is essential to ensure that urgent and life-threatening needs are attended to first. The prioritisation of care is a complex process which requires skill and expertise. It is also important to involve the person in the prioritisation of care. The nurse and person may have differing views on the prioritisation of care, and it is important to communicate and negotiate this. An example of this is found in Case study 3.1.

➡ Activity 3.15

Now spend some time reflecting on your own practice. Consider a time when a person's care had to be prioritised.

Person's needs:

1.

2.

3.

What did you do first?

Why did you choose to do things in this order?

When you have established the person's needs, it is possible to make a plan of care. It is usually most appropriate to devise a care plan. This provides documented evidence of the plan of care you have agreed with the person. It is then possible for all those involved in the care of that person to assist the person to meet his or her goals. An example of a person's goal is presented in Figure 3.4.

It should be noted that the goals identified for Mrs Smith (Figure 3.4) all meet the 'SMART' criteria. This means that goals should be:

- **Specific:** Goals should be precise, objective and explicit to the person and healthcare team.
- **Measurable:** There must be a clear way to measure whether the goal has been achieved. This may be a clinical sign (such as John's fluid intake will be 3000 mLs/day) or behaviour (such as Susan will be able to administer her insulin without supervision).
- **Achievable:** The goals must be achievable for the person based on his or her abilities and condition. There must also be adequate resources for the goal to be achieved.
- **Realistic:** Goals must be realistic for the individual. Unrealistic goals, which exceed the capability of the person, are purposeless and may lead to the person feeling demotivated.
- **Time-orientated:** Goals must have an allocated time frame by which they are measured. These may be short or long term.

Patient name: Sue Smith	
Hospital number: 1234567	
Date of birth: 01.02.1973	
Date: 21.05.2008	
Need/problem	**Signature**
Mrs Smith is confused and anxious regarding her recent diagnosis. Due to her anxiety she is tearful, unable to sleep and has a poor appetite.	
Goal	
For Mrs Smith to be able to demonstrate an understanding of her diagnosis and the treatment proposed	
For Mrs Smith to feel that all of her questions about her diagnosis have been answered	
For Mrs Smith's behaviour to demonstrate that she is less anxious through being less tearful, sleeping for longer periods and having an improved appetite	
Plan of care	**To be completed and reviewed by:**
Nursing team to communicate with Mrs Smith and provide information on her diagnosis	Ongoing throughout admission
Refer Mrs Smith to the clinical nurse specialist for a consultation	29.06.08
Provide information to Mrs Smith regarding available support groups and advice services	29.06.08
Provide written information leaflets for Mrs Smith to refer to and share with her family	29.06.08

Figure 3.4   Sample plan of care

Activity 3.16

Consider the person who you have cared for in practice. Using one of the needs that you have identified in the assessment process, devise a plan of care for the person in the blank care plan. Include some goals for the patient that meets the SMART criteria.

Patient name: Hospital number: Date of birth: Date:	
Need/problem	

(continued)

Activity 3.16 (*Continued*)

Patient name: Hospital number: Date of birth: Date:	
Goal	
Plan of care	To be completed and reviewed by:

It is also important to note that the goals set with a person may be short or long term. For example, a short-term goal for a person with learning disabilities may be to go to the shops accompanied by a key worker. However, a long-term goal may be to go to the shops and collect a list of items without assistance. Goals should, therefore, be reviewed regularly to establish whether they have been achieved. The evaluation of care will be discussed later in the chapter.

Principles of implementation of care

The implementation of care is concerned with delivering the plan of care identified in the second phase of the nursing process. As with all stages of the nursing process, this should involve the person as much as possible. In some situations, it may also be appropriate to involve the family or others in the implementation of care, if this is agreeable to the person. As a student nurse you are likely to be involved in the implementation of care for a number of individuals with very different goals. It is essential to only implement care which you are competent to give (Nursing and Midwifery Council, 2008). The implementation of care should be based on the best available research evidence to ensure that it is delivered in the most effective way. However, nurses may also draw upon their professional experience when considering the best way to implement care.

It is also important to consider who the best person is to implement the plan of care for a person. Wherever possible, it is desirable to encourage the person to take an active part in his or her own care. It is also often beneficial to involve a number of health professionals with differing expertise. For example, a person with a chest infection is likely to require the assistance of a physiotherapist who has expertise in methods to aid mucous clearance and improve lung function. It may also be appropriate to involve other people who have a significant role in the person's life. One example of this may be the involvement of a key worker for a person with learning disabilities who is admitted to hospital.

➡ Activity 3.17

Reflect on a recent practice experience, and identify those people involved in implementing a person's care in the table below.

Person involved in care implementation	Role

Principles of evaluation of care

When care has been implemented, it is essential that the effectiveness of that care is evaluated. The setting of measurable goals within the care plan should allow this process to happen. If goals have not been met, then it may be necessary to amend the way in which the care is delivered. For example, a goal may be set for a person at home to be able to independently prepare a meal. If the evaluation reveals that he or she is still unable to achieve this, it may be that the education or equipment provision was inappropriate to allow the person to achieve the goal. As with all stages of the nursing process, it is important to involve the person and those involved in the care in the evaluation process. It may be that the person's beliefs about the effectiveness of care differs from that of the nurse. Likewise, other professionals will make a valuable contribution to the process. If care has been effective, it may result in the achievement of the goal. This should then be documented in the care plan.

Following the evaluation stage, it is important that the person is reassessed. It may be that the needs identified in the original assessment have been met, or equally that new needs have emerged. For example, it may be that a person's initial goal was to be free from chest pain. This may have been achieved successfully, but the person may be suffering from nausea associated with the analgesia given. A revised plan of care would then need to be made in which a plan was identified to relieve the person's nausea.

The box below provides an example of how a person's care may be evaluated in their notes.

Date/Time: *01.02.2007 21.30*
Person details: *Elizabeth Smith*
Hospital number: *1234567*
Date of birth *02.04.1959*
Mrs Smith is pyrexial at 38.0°C. Blankets removed and oral Paracetamol administered. Vital signs recorded 2 hourly throughout the shift. Mrs Smith is now apyrexial at 36.0°C. Vital signs now to be recorded 4 hourly unless condition changes.

Signature:
Name:
Designation:

Activity 3.18

Think about the person for whom you devised a plan of care. Write an evaluation as if it may appear in their notes. Remember that your evaluation needs to report on the care that was given and the effectiveness of that care.

Factors affecting vital signs

There are many factors that may affect a person's vital signs including physical, social, psychological, environmental, procedure, medication, age and iatrogenic (caused inadvertently by a healthcare professional, intervention, treatment or diagnostic). For example, you may record the temperature of an older person and find it to be low at 35.0°C. However, you see in her notes that previously her temperature had been within normal limits. You realise that the lady is sitting by an open window and is not wearing her cardigan as usual. It is possible that the lady's temperature has been affected by environmental factors (a cold draft from the open window and inadequate clothing) rather than a biological cause. You would need to make adjustments to her environment.

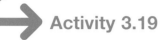 Activity 3.19

Write some examples of factors that may affect a person's vital signs.

Vital sign	Examples of factors affecting vital sign
Respiration	
Temperature	
Blood pressure	
Pulse	*Anxiety; such as a person who has just received information about their operation later that day.*

Now think about those vital signs you have measured and recorded in practice. Were there any recordings that you think deviated from the norm? If so, why?

Activity 3.20

Complete this section during your clinical placement.

	Vital sign recorded	Normal value	Person's vital sign	Possible reason for deviation
Person 1				
Person 2				
Person 3				
Person 4				
Person 5				

Deviations from the norm

It is important to know the normal values when monitoring vital signs. Some suggested normal values are presented in Table 3.1. However, it must be recognised that some people may normally function with vital signs that are outside of these ranges. For example, a very young healthy person may have a resting heart rate below 60 beats/min. It is also important to remember that different books and sources may give you different 'normal values' for vital signs. Always remember to look at what is 'normal' or usual for the person whom you are caring for.

Table 3.1   Normal values for vital signs

	Newborn	Childhood	Adulthood
Respiration rate/min	40–80	20–40 (Early childhood) 15–25 (Late childhood)	14–18 (Male) 16–20 (Female)
Temperature °C	36.0–37.5°C	36.0–37.5°C	36.0–37.5°C
Pulse Beats/min	120–160	1–12 months 80–140 12 months-2 years 80–130 2–6 years 75–120 6–12 years 75–110	60–100
Blood pressure mmHg	80/46	103/70	100/60–140/90

Documentation

Accurate documentation of all care given is a professional requirement. The Nursing and Midwifery Code states that 'you must ensure that the healthcare record for the patient or client is an accurate account of treatment, care planning and delivery' (Nursing and Midwifery Council, 2008). The documentation of vital signs is essential to provide a baseline set of data and to demonstrate trends in a person's condition. These must be recorded accurately and immediately following measurement. Most often the documentation of vital signs is completed in chart format to demonstrate the trends more clearly. The documentation of vital signs is also essential for effective communication with other members of the healthcare team.

You must ensure that you are familiar with local documentation guidelines in the area in which you are practicing. It is also important to supplement the observation chart with any other relevant assessment of the person. This may include other symptoms that he or she is experiencing. For example, a person with an altered respiratory rate may also show signs of shortness of breath, wheeze, coughing and so on. These enable healthcare professionals to make a more meaningful and informed assessment of the person.

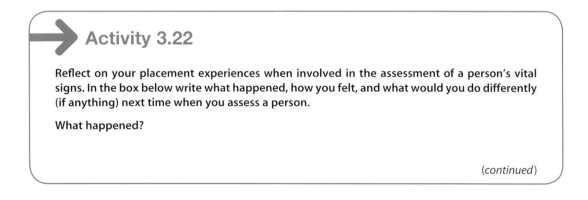

Activity 3.21

What are the key considerations when completing patient documentation?

You may also wish to read the *Guidelines for Records and Record Keeping* (Nursing and Midwifery Council, 2005). In addition to documenting the vital signs, it is also important to document the care planned and any action taken. For example, if a person is hypertensive (has elevated blood pressure) you may administer medication to reduce this. It is important to evaluate the treatment by reassessing the person's vital signs and to document the findings. This provides a written record of the nursing care and allows the effectiveness of care to be recorded.

Activity 3.22

Reflect on your placement experiences when involved in the assessment of a person's vital signs. In the box below write what happened, how you felt, and what would you do differently (if anything) next time when you assess a person.

What happened?

(continued)

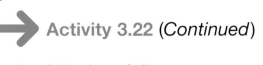

Activity 3.22 (*Continued*)

How did it make you feel?

What would you do differently (if anything) next time?

Case Studies: Consider the case studies below and discuss some of the issues with your mentor or supervisor at work. You can also find some suggested answers on the website.

Case study 3.1

A lady is admitted to an acute mental health setting following an exacerbation of paranoid schizophrenia. She is known to be at risk of harming herself or others. Your first priority is to maintain a safe environment for the lady and those around her. However, during your assessment the lady tells you that she is most concerned about her cats that have been left at home. She identifies that one of her immediate needs is to ensure that arrangements are made to care for them.

It is important to recognise that you and the lady have identified different priorities within the plan of care. You must acknowledge the need she has expressed and communicate your understanding. However, you are also required to communicate the importance of maintaining her safety and ensure that care is planned to meet this need as a priority. This is because there is potential for harm to occur to the lady and others.

Case study 3.2

Consider this scenario. Think about the possible effects you might see when taking this gentleman's vital signs.

You visit an elderly gentleman in his own home during the winter, and have been asked to assess and record his vital signs. The gentleman is in the garden when you arrive and rushes in to greet you. He is anxious that you are a few minutes late for the appointment. What effect would you expect this activity to have on his vital signs?

Case study 3.3

Mrs Smith is an 80-year-old lady who is admitted to the medical assessment unit where you are working. You are asked to complete her initial assessment and devise a plan of care. Mrs Smith has been admitted by ambulance following a 4-day history of feeling unwell. Mrs Smith tells you that she has had chronic obstructive pulmonary disease (COPD) for approximately 10 years. Over the past 4 days, she has felt increasingly breathless and tired. As you are talking with her, you notice that she is unable to complete full sentences without drawing a breath. She has been resting in bed for the past 2 days. Her appetite has been poor, and she has been too breathless to prepare and eat a meal. She has been unable to walk to the shop as usual to collect her shopping. Her family does not live locally, and have just been informed of her admission to hospital. During the assessment, Mrs Smith becomes upset as she is concerned about her 2 cats that are at home. Mrs Smith reports that she has started to cough and has been producing green sputum.

As part of the initial assessment you measure and record Mrs Smith's vital signs which are:

Respiratory rate: 31; temperature: 38.1; pulse 108 (weak); blood pressure: 85/54.

Chapter summary

This chapter has introduced the principles of assessing, planning, implementing and evaluating care which is known as the nursing process. One key area of assessment is the assessment of vital signs which provide an indication of the state of core physical functions. The most commonly recorded vital signs are respiratory rate, temperature, pulse and blood pressure. It is important to remember that these measurements may be affected by a number of physical, emotional and environmental factors. Measurements should be taken and recorded accurately. However, the assessment of a person includes other important information which may relate to the person's physical, psychological, social, emotional and spiritual well-being. Many different tools are available in practice to aid assessment. The thorough assessment of a person allows appropriate care to be planned. Wherever possible, care should be planned in partnership with the person. A care plan is a most appropriate way of setting a person's goals which should fulfil the SMART criteria. Care can then be implemented to enable the person to meet his or her goals. Following the implementation of care, it is important to evaluate the effectiveness of the care delivered. It is then necessary to return to the care plan to see if goals have been achieved and if changes should be made to the planned care. Throughout all phases of the nursing process, it is vital to maintain accurate and detailed documentation which is a requirement of professional practice.

Answers to Activities

Activity 3.1 Key terms

Use your nursing dictionary to look up the following terms and provide a complete definition of each term.

Term	Definition
Tachypnoeic	Abnormally rapid rate of breathing
Bradypnoeic	Abnormally slow rate of breathing
Apnoeic	Cessation of breathing
Tachycardic	Fast heart beat, usually greater than 90 beats/min
Bradycardic	Slow heart beat, usually less than 60 beats/min
Hypertensive	High blood pressure
Hypotensive	Low blood pressure
Pyrexial	Rise of body temperature, usually between 37 and 40°C
Apyrexial	Temperature within normal limits
Hyperthermic	Exceedingly high body temperature
Hypothermic	Exceedingly low body temperature

Activity 3.2

Make a note of some of your thoughts. For example, you may have tried to record a person's vital signs but felt very anxious about explaining your findings to the person.

Activity 3.3

Write down some of the key considerations when assessing a person's respiratory rate.

● Ensure that the person is comfortable and has not undergone recent exercise as this could adversely affect the respiratory rate.
● Measure respiratory rate for 60 s.

Activity 3.3 (*Continued*)

- It may be useful to carry out respiratory rate assessment immediately after checking radial pulse. If the nurse still has finger on radial pulse site, it appears to the person as if the nurse is still checking the pulse. This reduces the person's awareness and the likelihood of the respiratory rate being affected.
- Observing for other signs of respiratory effort such as pursed lips, nasal flaring, use of accessory muscles (muscles other than the diaphragm and intercostal muscles which are used when breathing becomes laboured).
- Record the respiratory rate accurately in the person's notes.
- Observe for trends in the person's vital signs.
- Report abnormalities to a qualified practitioner.

Activity 3.4

Identify some of the advantages and disadvantages of using these four recording sites.

	Advantages	Disadvantages
Oral	<ul><li>Easily accessible</li><li>Changes in core temperature are quickly reflected in sublingual pockets due to rapid response of thermoreceptors</li></ul>	<ul><li>Temperature may be affected by ingested foods and drink, smoking, increased respiratory rate</li><li>Probe must be in sublingual pocket and not in area in front of the tongue</li><li>May be dangerous in a person who is confused, at risk of seizures or has an altered level of consciousness</li></ul>
Rectal	<ul><li>More accurate indication of core temperature than oral site as it is protected from the environment</li></ul>	<ul><li>Invasive and may be unacceptable to the person</li><li>Risk of bowel perforation if used in children</li><li>Soft stool in bowel may affect reading</li></ul>
Axillary	<ul><li>Useful for people who are unsuitable to use other sites</li></ul>	<ul><li>Less accurate than oral and rectal sites</li><li>May result in variation if different axilla is used</li></ul>
Tympanic membrane	<ul><li>Often easy to access and non-invasive</li></ul>	<ul><li>Potential inaccurate readings due to incorrect</li></ul>

(continued)

Activity 3.4 (*Continued*)

	Advantages	Disadvantages
	• Correlates well with core temperature as tympanic membrane shares the same arterial blood supply as the hypothalamus (Gallimore, 2004)	placement of probe, damaged probe lens, insufficient time between readings

Activity 3.5

Label the pulse points below.

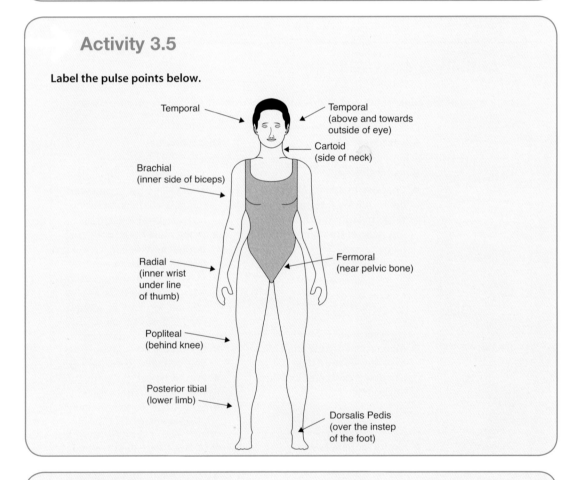

Temporal

Temporal
(above and towards
outside of eye)

Cartoid
(side of neck)

Brachial
(inner side of biceps)

Radial
(inner wrist
under line
of thumb)

Fermoral
(near pelvic bone)

Popliteal
(behind knee)

Posterior tibial
(lower limb)

Dorsalis Pedis
(over the instep
of the foot)

Activity 3.6

Reflect on your practice and record the sites you have used to measure a person's pulse and the reasons why this might have been.

Activity 3.7

Reflect on taking a person's radial pulse and the considerations you would make.

- Ensure that the person is at rest and has not recently undertaken exercise.
- Explain the procedure to the person.
- Obtain the person's consent.
- Ensure that the person is comfortable.
- Use first, second or third finger to press gently. This is because the thumb and forefinger have pulses and these may be mistaken for the person's pulse.
- Count for 60 s.
- If the pulse appears irregular, it may be necessary make a more detailed assessment of the person. This may include an electrocardiogram (ECG), apex pulse recording and so on.
- Record the pulse accurately in the person's notes.
- Observe for trends in the person's vital signs.
- Report abnormalities to a qualified practitioner.

Activity 3.8

Label the diagram of the heart.

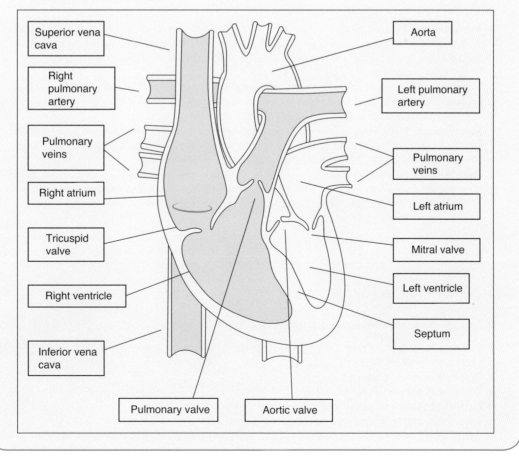

Activity 3.9

Define these two terms and identify the related physiology.

	Definition
Systolic	The maximum pressure which occurs after ventricular contraction (systole). This is therefore the pressure in the *contracting* phase.
Diastolic	The minimum pressure to which arterial pressure has fallen before the next ventricular systole. This is therefore the pressure in the *resting* phase (diastole). For a more detailed explanation of the physiology of blood pressure, see Montague *et al.* (2005).

Activity 3.10

Label the equipment shown in the figure below. Try to list the purpose of each part of the equipment.

a. **Manometer:** This part of the system is usually filled with mercury and provides the blood pressure reading based on the sounds heard. It should be placed on a flat surface and must be visible at eye level. Special care must be taken with mercury devices, particularly in the event of spillages or disposal.

b. **Inflation bulb, control valve and rubber tubing:** These parts allow the cuff to be inflated and air to be released in a controlled manner from the system. It must be checked for leaks and cracks to avoid inaccuracies.

c. **Stethoscope:** This is used to listen to the appearance and disappearance of the sounds related to blood pressure (Korotkoff's sounds). The diaphragm of the stethoscope should be placed directly over the pulse point of the brachial artery.

d. **Cuff:** This part is wrapped around the arm enclosing the inflatable rubber bladder. It is essential that the cuff covers 80% of the circumference of the arm and that the centre of the bladder covers the brachial artery (Dougherty and Lister, 2008). These may either be washable or suitable for single patient use.

Activity 3.11

Make a list of the key considerations whilst taking a blood pressure.

- Ensure that the person is at rest and has not recently undertaken exercise.
- Explain the procedure to the person.
- Obtain the person's consent.
- Ensure that the person is comfortable.
- Check all equipment is available and in good repair.
- Ensure that tight clothing around the arm is removed.
- Ensure accurate positioning of all equipment including cuff, stethoscope and manometer.

Activity 3.11 (*Continued*)

- Estimate systolic pressure first using radial pulse (see Dougherty and Lister, 2008).
- Clean equipment after use.
- Record the blood pressure accurately in the person's notes.
- Observe for trends in the person's vital signs.
- Report abnormalities to a qualified practitioner.

Activity 3.12

Write down some examples of assessment tools that you have seen used in practice.

- Pain assessment tools
- Anxiety and depression scale
- Pressure risk assessment tools
- Mini-mental state examination
- Nutrition assessment tools
- Family assessment tools
- Special education assessment tools

Activity 3.13

Think about the assessments you have seen in practice and list some of the skills that you used.

- Listening
- Observing
- Verbal communication
- Use of open and closed questions
- Non-verbal communication
- Physical examination
- Measurements

Activity 3.14

Write an example of a closed and open question. Think about the types of response do you think each would elicit.

Closed question   "Are you alright Mr Jones?"

Open question   "Mr Jones, tell me about your pain at the moment."

Activity 3.15

Now spend some time reflecting on your own practice. Consider a time when a person's care had to be prioritised.

Person's needs:

1.

2.

3.

What did you do first?

Why did you choose to do things in this order?
This is personal to you and your practice. You can discuss this with your mentor or supervisor.

Activity 3.16

Consider the person who you have cared for in practice. Using one of the needs that you have identified in the assessment process, devise a plan of care for the person in the blank care plan. Include some goals for the patient that meets the SMART criteria.

Patient name: Hospital number: Date of birth: Date:	
Need/problem	
Goal	
Plan of care	To be completed and reviewed by:

This is personal to you and your practice. You can discuss this with your mentor or supervisor.

Activity 3.17

Reflect on a recent practice experience, and identify those people involved in implementing a person's care in the table below.

Person involved in care implementation	Role
Nurse	
Doctor	
Physiotherapist	
Health Care Assistant	
Tissue Viability Nurse	

Activity 3.18

Think about the person for whom you devised a plan of care. Write an evaluation as if it may appear in their notes. Remember that your evaluation needs to report on the care that was given and the effectiveness of that care.

Mrs Jones has complained of pain in her sacrum today. Pain relief given at 10 AM with good effect. Following assessment of her wound, it was noted that the skin was broken. Dressing applied and wound nurse contacted. Wound superficial with bleeding around the edges. Patient pyrexial 39°. Antipyretic last given at 2 PM with good effect. Commenced hourly vital signs. Mrs Jones is very anxious, reassurance given. Nursed on left side, for 2 hourly turns overnight.
Sign and date (don't forget this bit!)

Activity 3.19

Write some examples of factors that may affect a person's vital signs.

Vital sign	Examples of factors affecting vital sign
Respiration	✓ Emotional stress/excitement/anxiety ✓ Exercise ✓ Existing respiratory condition such as bronchiectasis or asthma ✓ Infection ✓ Pain ✓ Long-standing smoker ✓ Medications such as analgesics and sedatives may reduce respiratory rate ✓ Injury to brainstem where respiratory centre is located ✓ Other causes of reduced consciousness such as post seizure, intoxication and so on

(continued)

Activity 3.19 (Continued)

Vital sign	Examples of factors affecting vital sign
Temperature	✓ Daily fluctuations. Temperature higher in the evening than in the morning ✓ Eating/drinking hot/cold fluids and foods ✓ Exercise ✓ Ovulation ✓ Environmental temperature particularly for older and young people. You may have seen this in a person who lives in a cold environment or someone who has undergone surgery ✓ Infection ✓ Medication ✓ Central nervous system damage such as stroke, head injury
Blood pressure	✓ Fluid imbalance ✓ Medication ✓ Emotional stress/excitement/anxiety ✓ Renal disease ✓ Pain
Pulse	✓ Dehydration ✓ Fluid loss (hypovolaemia) ✓ Exercise ✓ Emotional stress/excitement/anxiety ✓ Incompatible blood transfusion ✓ Medication such as salbutamol may increase pulse ✓ Medication such as digoxin, sedatives may decrease pulse ✓ Infection ✓ Cerebral insult ✓ Pain

Activity 3.20

Complete this section during your clinical placement.

	Vital sign recorded	Normal value	Person's vital sign	Possible reason for deviation
Person 1				
Person 2				
Person 3				
Person 4				
Person 5				

Activity 3.21

What are the key considerations when completing patient documentation?

- Ensure person's name, date of birth and identification number appears on all documentation.
- Write clearly in black ink.
- Avoid subjective terms such as 'feeling unwell'. Avoid jargon and offensive or subjective statements.
- Use only approved abbreviations.
- Ensure that you sign, date and print your name on all entries.
- Sign all entries and print signature alongside first entry.

Activity 3.22

Reflect on your placement experiences when involved in the assessment of a person's vital signs. In the box below write what happened, how you felt, and what would you do differently (if anything) next time when you assess a person.

What happened?

- Describe the scenario briefly relating to your learning need.

How did it make you feel?

- Did you feel good or bad about it?
- What was good or bad about the situation?
- Did you have adequate underpinning knowledge to carry out the care?
- If you had previous experience of similar situation, was it useful this time?

What would you do differently (if anything) next time?

- Has this personal experience prepared you to do further reading and gained more practice under supervision?

This is only a guide. Please address the sub-headings to meet your own learning needs.

References

Butler-Williams, C. (2005) Increasing staff awareness of respiratory rate significance. *Nursing Times* **101** (27), 35–37.

Carroll, M. (2000) An evaluation of temperature measurement. *Nursing Standard* **14** (44), 39–43.

Castledine, G. (2006) The importance of measuring and recording vital signs correctly. *British Journal of Nursing* **15** (5), 285.

Chellel, A. Fraser, J., Fender, V., Higgs, D., Buras-Rees, S., Hook, L., *et al.* (2002) Nursing observations on ward: patients at risk of critical illness. *Nursing Times* **98** (46), 36–39.

Cork, A. (2007) Theory and practice of manual blood pressure measurement. *Nursing Standard* **22** (14–16), 47–50.

Department of Health (2001) *National Service Framework for Older People* (London: HMSO).

Department of Health (2003) *Essence of care. Patient-focused benchmarks for clinical governance* (London: NHS Modernisation Agency).

Dougherty, L. and Lister, S. (2008) *The Royal Marsden Hospital Manual of Clinical Nursing Procedures,* 7th edn (Oxford: Blackwell).

Eşer, I., Khorshid, L., Güneş, U. and Demir, Y. (2006) The effect of different body positions on blood pressure. *Journal of Clinical Nursing* **16**, 137–140.

Gallimore, D. (2004) Reviewing the effectiveness of tympanic thermometers. *Nursing Times* **100** (32), 32–34.

Hinckley, P. and Walker, S. (2005) Measuring blood pressure. *New Practice Nurse* **29** (9), 54–56.

Hodgetts, T.J., Kenward, G., Vlachonikolis, I.G., Payne, S. and Castle, N. (2002) The identification of risk factors for cardiac arrest and formulation of activation criteria to alert a medical emergency team. *Resuscitation* **54** (2), 125–131.

Hogston, R. and Marjoram, B. (2007) *Foundations of Nursing Practice. Leading the Way* (Basingstoke: Palgrave Macmillan).

Jamieson, L.M., Whyte, L.A. and McCall, J.M. (2007) *Clinical Nursing Practices*, 5th edn (London: Churchill Livingstone).

Kenward, G. (2001) Time to put the R back in TPR. *Nursing Times* **97** (32), 32–33.

Kenworthy, N., Snowley, G. and Gilling, C. (2002) *Common Foundations Studies in Nursing*, 3rd edn (London: Churchill Livingstone).

Kisiel, M. and Perkins, C. (2006) Nursing observations: knowledge to help prevent critical illness. *British Journal of Nursing* **15** (19), 1052–1056.

Kozier, B., Erb, G., Berman, A., Snyder, S., Lake, R. and Harvey, S. (2008) *Fundamentals of Nursing. Concepts, Process and Practice* (Harlow: Pearson Education).

McAlister, F. and Straus, S. (2001) Measurement of blood pressure: an evidence based review. *British Medical Journal* **322**, 908–911.

McArthur-Rouse, F. (2001) Critical care outreach services and early warning scoring systems: a review of the literature. *Journal of Advanced Nursing* **36**, 696–704.

Montague, S.E, Watson, R. and Herbert, R. (2005) *Physiology for Nursing Practice*, 5th edn (London: Bailliere Tindall).

Nursing and Midwifery Council (2005) *Guidelines for Records and Record Keeping* (London: Nursing and Midwifery Council).

Nursing and Midwifery Council (2008) *The Code: Standards of Conduct, Performance and Ethics for Nurses and Midwives* (London: Nursing and Midwifery Council).

O'Brien, E., Asmar, R., Bellin, L., *et al.* (2003) European society of hypertension recommendations for conventional, ambulatory and home blood pressure measurement. *Journal of Hypertension* **21** (5), 821–848.

Resuscitation Council UK (2005) *Prevention of In-Hospital Cardiac Arrest and Decisions About Cardiopulmonary Resuscitation* (London: Resuscitation Council UK).

Simpson, M.C. (2006) Traceable calibration for blood pressure and temperature monitoring. *Nursing Standard* **22** (21), 42–47.

Trim, J. (2005) Monitoring temperature. *Nursing Times* **101**, (20), 30–31.

Wallymahmed, M. (2008) Blood pressure measurement. *Nursing Standard* **22** (19), 45–48.

Waterlow, J. (2005) Pressure ulcer risk assessment and prevention. http://www.judy-waterlow.co.uk/ (accessed 17 July 2008).

Werntoft, E., Edberg, A., Rooke, L., Hermerén, G., Elmståhl, S. and Hallberg, I. (2005). Older people's views of prioritization in health care. The applicability of an interview study. *International Journal of Older People Nursing* **14**, 64–74.

Further reading

Alexander, M., Fawcett, J. and Runciman, P. (2006) *Nursing Practice. Hospital and Home*, 3rd edn (Edinburgh: Churchill Livingstone).

Brooker, C. and Waugh, A. (2007) *Foundations of Nursing Practice- Fundamentals of Holistic Care* (London: Elsevier Moby).

Heath, B.M. (1995) *Potter and Perry's Foundations in Nursing Theory and Practice* (London: Mosby).

National Institute for Health and Clinical Excellence (2003) *Triage, Assessment, Investigation and Early Management of Head Injury in Infants, Children and Adults* (London: NICE).

Richardson, M. (2003) Physiology for practice: the mechanisms controlling respiration. *Nursing Times* **99** (48), 48–50.

Stevenson, T. (2004) Achieving best practice in routine observation of hospital patients. *Nursing Times* **100** (34), 34–35.

Walsh, M. and Crumbie, A. (2007) *Watson's Clinical Nursing and Related Sciences*, 7th edn (London. Baillière Tindall).

Watson, D. (2006) The impact of accurate patient assessment on quality care. *Nursing Times* **102** (34), 34–37.

Weller, B. (2005) *Bailliere's Nurses' Dictionary*, 24th edn (London: Baillière Tindall).

4 Principles of respiratory care

VIJAYA RAJOO NAIDU AND LOUISE LAWSON

Aims

The aim of this chapter is to introduce you to the key principles of respiratory care and provide an overview of the factors that influence respiration.

Learning objectives

On completion of this chapter, you will learn to:

- Describe the fundamental process of respiration
- Recognise some pre-disposing factors that can influence normal respiration
- Recognise barriers to communication during altered respiration
- Acknowledge the importance of privacy and dignity when nursing patients with respiratory conditions
- Start discussing appropriate care plans to achieve the goals in respiratory assessment
- Document respiratory assessment accurately
- Demonstrate an ability to use commonly required equipment when assessing respiration such as peak flow meter and pulse oximetry

Introduction

There are numerous resources available concerning nursing observation of patients and each one never fails to emphasise the significance of performing and recording of vital signs accurately. Nursing observation of a patient is an acquired skill attained by understanding the knowledge underpinning practice that is enhanced over the years. The assessment of the respiratory system is unique and as important as the rest of the patient's vital sign observation and care. Chellel *et al.* (2002) highlighted that the respiratory rate of a patient is often poorly documented and something that is taken for granted when there are approximately 8 million people in the UK who suffer from lung disease (Whyte, 2004). To omit respiratory assessment is considered poor practice and can be seen as clinical negligence when other vital signs are within normal range. The monitoring and assessment of the respiratory system is crucial to ascertain whether life is sustainable or not and is directly related to the cardio pulmonary resuscitation (CPR) principle. To understand the underpinning theory of respiratory system, monitoring and assessment is essential; therefore, gaining some knowledge of the anatomy and physiology of the respiratory system is essential before attempting to gain any experience in performing the skill correctly.

This chapter will help you to gain knowledge in performing the monitoring and assessment of respiratory system. This chapter prepares you as pre-qualified nurses or other healthcare professionals to build confidence during your education or interim period to achieve competence (NMC, 2008). The discussion and activities included in this chapter will address respiratory observation skills, assessment and health promotion. Issues surrounding communication, privacy, dignity, health and safety will be discussed. Furthermore, you can reflect on past experiences of caring for someone with respiratory difficulties and relate these to the discussions and activities within this chapter. The answers to the activities can be found at the end of the chapter. Additionally, you are encouraged to read related local health policies on infection control and find out about the use of medical equipment and portable oxygen apparatus for both hospital and community settings.

Self-assessment

Let us explore how you would feel when you witness someone with respiratory difficulties such as breathlessness. Write down whatever comes to your mind in the stars below and let us work on how to overcome them as we work through this chapter. Only practice, experience and knowledge would help you to develop from a novice, advanced beginner, competent, proficient to expert status (Benner, 1984) because these different levels reflect changes in development of skilled performance.

Activity 4.1 Your thoughts on witnessing someone with respiratory difficulties

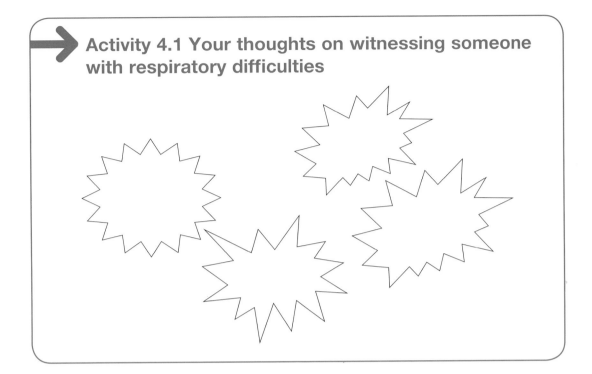

Assessment of respiration

It is important to understand the terminology related to vital signs, especially observation of respiration. You may be familiar with some of the terms and others you may need to find out. Please use a nurse's dictionary to help define the terms related to respiratory conditions.

Activity 4.2 Key terms

Term	Definition
Tachypnoea	
Bradypnoea	
Apnoea	
Eupnoea	
Cheyne–Stokes	
Stridor	

(continued)

Activity 4.2 (Continued)

Term	Definition
Respiration	
Oxygen saturation	
Peak flow	
Cyanosis	
Orthopnoea	

Monitoring of vital signs includes observation of respiratory physiological measurements that may be influenced by physical, emotional and environmental factors. Respiration, pulse rate, temperature and blood pressure data are important to implement and evaluate care as changes can occur. Some of these physiological changes may be potentially life threatening. The most common method to measure respiration is the fundamental observation of the patient's chest for equal movement to determine that it is bilateral and symmetrical (Bennett, 2002).

Activity 4.3

When would you monitor a patient's respiratory rate?

Patient assessment

During respiratory assessment, the patient's general appearance, posture, presenting complaints, past medical history, social history and observation of physical symptoms are crucial (Bennett, 2003). This information prompts the implementation of appropriate care and evaluation of its effectiveness. When observing the patient's appearance, focus on the colour of lips, skin and finger nails looking for cyanosis, facial flushing, cold, warm, clammy or dry skin, shape and movement of chest wall. Appearance also includes patients' level of consciousness; for instance, are they alert, confused, agitated, anxious, exhausted, in pain or unresponsive? However, posture may relate to localised areas of pain, fear and orthopnoea suggesting difficulty in breathing or general discomfort (Bennett, 2002).

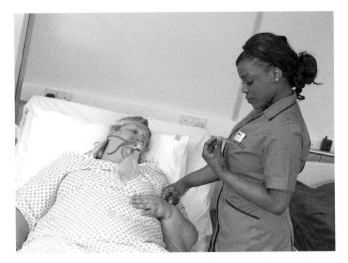

Figure 4.1   Counting respirations at the same time as the pulse

Cyanosis is a late sign when there is low oxygenated haemoglobin level (Hb less than 5 mg/dl) in the blood or hypoxia with saturation as low as less than 80% (Woodrow, 2002). Cyanosis can be peripheral or central. Peripheral cyanosis is noticeable in the skin, nail bed, earlobes, mouth and finger tips by a tinge of bluish purple discolouration (Casey, 2001). This is due to vasoconstriction and stasis of blood in the extremities and increased oxygenation extraction by peripheral tissues. In central cyanosis, the tongue and lips are slightly dusky and bluish grey in colour indicating an acute sign of hypoxia or respiratory disease (Jevon and Ewens, 2001).

It is common practice to measure respiratory rate when pulse rate is monitored without removing the fingers over the chosen artery to prevent alerting patient where the reading can be altered (Wilkins *et al.*, 2005) (see Figure 4.1). In Activity 4.3, you might have considered monitoring respiratory rate on arrival or before admission of a patient or before the start of a procedure or pre-operatively to act as baseline of the respiratory system (Kenward, 2001). When a patient's condition deteriorates or improves, the recordings help to evaluate care.

You will need to report any abnormalities to your mentor or a qualified nurse.

Respiratory rate is observed as a baseline, after surgery, during treatment, for example, when on a morphine infusion (an overdose of morphine depresses the respiratory centre in the brain), or for monitoring a response to treatment or medication.

In order to perform a full respiratory assessment, it is mandatory to understand the respiratory system; see Figure 4.2. Firstly, refer to any anatomy and physiology textbook to review the respiratory system and complete Activity 4.4.

Activity 4.4

Using an anatomy and physiology textbook, label the diagram in Figure 4.2, then write down the function of each section of the respiratory system.

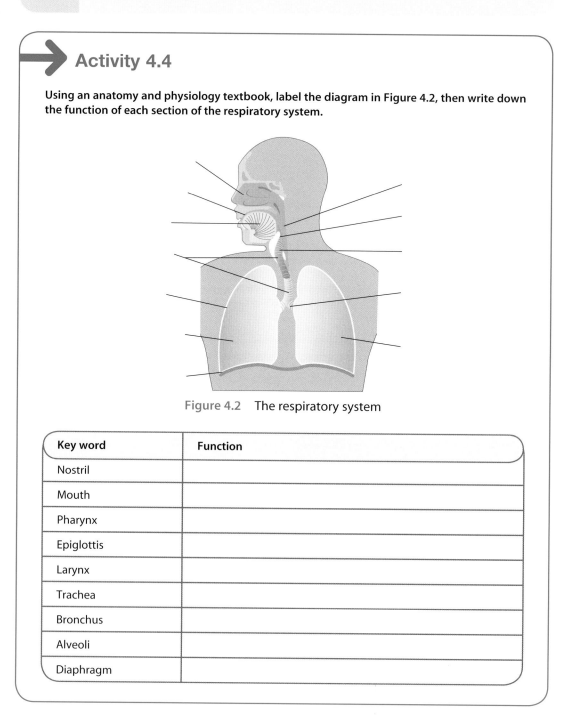

Figure 4.2   The respiratory system

Key word	Function
Nostril	
Mouth	
Pharynx	
Epiglottis	
Larynx	
Trachea	
Bronchus	
Alveoli	
Diaphragm	

The respiratory system focuses on breathing where oxygen (O_2) is supplied and carbon dioxide (CO_2) is removed. This is achieved by inspiration (breathing in) when oxygen is inhaled and expiration (breathing out) when carbon dioxide is exhaled. Therefore, respiration includes both inspiration and expiration. The changes in oxygen and carbon dioxide can alter normal breathing where the respiratory system compensates readily. When performing a respiratory assessment, the rate is commonly performed as standard; however, pattern, depth, breath sounds and oxygen saturation can also be included depending on the condition of the patient.

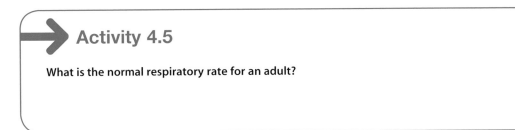

Activity 4.5

What is the normal respiratory rate for an adult?

Sometimes, it is necessary to expose a patient's chest, especially during acute illness or emergency, to observe the rise and fall of the chest wall, and to monitor the use of accessory muscles or carry out treatment (Moore, 2007).

It is every healthcare professional's responsibility to respect and maintain the patient's privacy and dignity at all times in any NHS healthcare trust (DH, 2001).

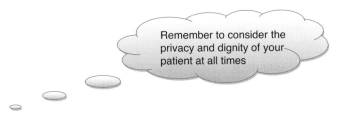

Remember to consider the privacy and dignity of your patient at all times

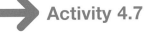

Activity 4.6

Describe what you understand by respiratory pattern.

Activity 4.7

Outline the factors that are important when assessing respiratory depth.

Table 4.1   Respiratory rate of different age groups
(*Source:* Adapted from Glasper *et al.* (2007)).

Age	Respiratory rate (breaths/min)
Neonate	60–80
1 year	30–40
1–2 years	25–35
2–5 years	25–30
5–12 years	20–25
Adult	15–20
Athlete	12–20

Respiratory rate is the number of respiratory cycles in 1 min. The respiratory cycle includes inspiration and expiration. Normal respiration is quiet, about 12–18 breaths per minute in an adult (Ahern and Phipot, 2002). Respiratory rates vary according to age, size, gender and condition of patient. For the respiratory rate of different age groups, see Table 4.1. When the respiratory rate exceeds the normal rate, it is called **tachypnoea**. However, it is abnormal at any age to have tachypnoea more than 60 breaths per minute (Wilkins *et al.*, 2005).

Activity 4.8

During a respiratory assessment of a patient, you notice that the patient is tachypnoeic and you wonder why there is an increase in his or her respiratory rate.

List below some factors that could cause tachypnoea.

-
-
-
-
-
-
-

It is the normal body's response to be **tachypnoeic** when a person experiences stress, fear, exercise, fever, anxiety, pain, low oxygen in the arterial system and metabolic acidosis (Wilkins *et al.*, 2005). Changes in environmental temperature can also influence respiratory rate. In deep sleep, the respiratory rate falls to its lowest normal level (Baillie, 2005). **Bradypnoea** is referred to as decreased respiratory rate. Although bradypnoea is rare, it may be the result of drug overdose or as a side effect of medications such as narcotics (Wilkins *et al.*, 2005), in head injuries or hypothermia. If there is absence of respiration, it is referred to as **apnoea**.

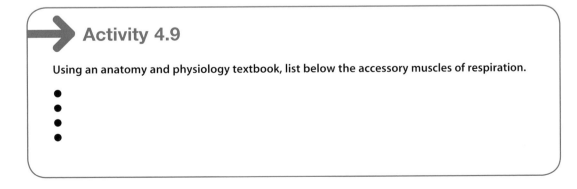

Next time you undertake a respiratory assessment, monitor the respiratory rate, then observe for any sounds by placing your stethoscope on your patient's chest.

Respiratory pattern and effort refer to the rhythm of breathing. A healthy adult at rest has minimal effort on inhalation and exhalation with a consistent rate (Wilkins *et al.*, 2005). The **inspiratory** and **expiratory** (I/E) phases determine the respiratory pattern. The regularity, duration and effort applied during each inhalation and exhalation provide vital indications as to the type of respiratory problem the patient may present. The breathing pattern can be rapid and shallow due to low lung volume with increased respiratory rate, which can be seen in patients with restrictive lung disease such as chronic obstructive pulmonary disease (COPD). Normal I/E ratio is 1:1. An asthmatic patient has prolonged exhalation time, may be 1:3 or 1:4 I/E ratio (Wilkins *et al.*, 2005).

When breathing is difficult or laboured, it is called **dyspnoea**. Patients may use their accessory muscles of respiration to facilitate effort and increase lung volume. Some patients may express shortness of breath as they cannot get enough air into their lungs (Karnani *et al.*, 2005). When patients are **dyspnoeic**, they often tend to breathe through their mouth rather than nose due to less resistance to airflow in the mouth and this can cause mouth dryness. Here, you must consider the necessity of oral hygiene to maintain moist oral cavity (Baillie, 2005). The terms shortness of breath, breathlessness and dyspnoea all imply difficulty in breathing (Bozkurt and Mann, 2003) and the causes are related to different problems in the body (see Table 4.2), but, prolonged and severe dyspnoea can cause exhaustion and respiratory arrest (Woodrow, 2002).

Activity 4.9

Using an anatomy and physiology textbook, list below the accessory muscles of respiration.

-
-
-
-

Table 4.2   Causes of breathlessness
(*Source:* Adapted from Bennett, 2003).

Cause	Symptoms
Obstructive disorders of the airway	Narrowed and obstructed airways due to excessive secretion, aspiration of foreign body/fluid or tumour, compression by enlarged lymph nodes/tumours and destruction of lung tissue
Restrictive disorders	Limited lung expansion and reduced lung volumes due to stiffness of chest wall, malfunction of respiratory muscles, accumulation of fluid/air/blood in the pleural cavity and consolidation of lung tissue
Pulmonary vascular disorders	Pulmonary vascular disease results from pulmonary hypertension, pulmonary oedema and pulmonary embolism
Infection	Viral or bacterial infection or aspiration of gastric content or retention of respiratory secretions
Trauma	As a result of crushing, penetrating or compression injuries to chest
Systemic illness problems	May be cardiac, metabolic, reduced oxygen-carrying capacity, toxic inhalation, depression of respiratory centre and drugs such as opiates suppresses the central nervous system
Pregnancy	The diaphragm misplaces as the uterus enlarges in the third trimester and may affect lung expansion (Moore, 2007)

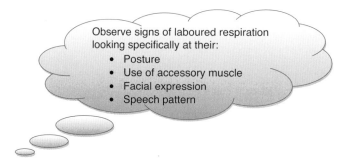

Observe signs of laboured respiration looking specifically at their:
- Posture
- Use of accessory muscle
- Facial expression
- Speech pattern

During dyspnoea, the patients cannot lie flat as they struggle for their breath, so easier breathing is best achieved in upright or crouched-forward positions (Bennett, 2003). It is good practice to support the patients well with pillows, as they need to be sitting up in bed or in an armchair to facilitate maximum breathing. There are some people who cannot breathe unless they are upright and this is referred to as **orthopnoea**.

Respiratory depth can be either shallow or deep with rapid or slow breathing. The respiratory depth can be made easy by observation or feeling the chest movement or listening to breath sounds with a stethoscope (Bennett, 2003). When respiration is rapid and deep (e.g. during a panic attack), this is called **hyperventilation** where carbon dioxide is low and can result in dizziness and fainting due to cerebral vasoconstriction (Baillie, 2005). With hyperventilating patients, you can help to reassure the patients and advise them to breathe in and out of a paper bag (re-breath exhaled air is rich in carbon dioxide) to restore normal levels.

Slow and shallow breathing is referred to as **hypoventilation** where gas exchange is poor. Only the upper part of the lung supports shallow breathing and rest of the lung remains warm and moist, promoting bacterial growth that can result in chest infection (Woodrow, 2002). It is important to observe for equal expansion of both sides of the chest, especially in chest injury. Apnoea could occur during hypoventilation and breathing may resume when the carbon dioxide level is high. **Cheyne–Stokes** respiration refers to irregular breathing (hyperventilation) with periods of apnoea lasting approximately 15–20 s (Wilkins *et al.*, 2005) resulting from left ventricular failure or cerebral injury and often at the end stage of life (Moore, 2007). Rapid and deep ventilation is termed as **Kussmaul's respiration** and is common in people with severe acidosis (Kennedy, 2007). The patient feels the urge to breathe deeply (air hunger); this is entirely involuntary. Kussmaul originally identified this type of breathing as a sign of coma and imminent death in patients with diabetes.

Respiratory sounds can be heard with or without a stethoscope (**auscultation**). During normal breathing, it is quiet, without using a stethoscope. It is not normal to be able to hear audible breath sounds, especially without a stethoscope. Respiratory sounds such as **wheeze**, **stridor** and snoring are a few of the common abnormal breath sounds (see Table 4.3).

Table 4.3   Breath sounds and how they are associated with the closest anatomical structures

Breath sounds (Wilkins *et al.*, 2005)	
Wheeze	Audible musical sound pronounced on expiration, in asthma, chronic bronchitis, emphysema
Rhonchi	Identified on auscultation, similar to wheeze
Stridor	High-pitched sound occurring on inspiration in upper airway caused by tracheal or laryngeal obstruction
Crackles	Identified on auscultation during inspiration
Absent	Common in emphysema, pleural effusion

A wheeze is often heard in people with **asthma** when air is forced through narrowed respiratory passages during expiration. A **stridor** is heard in **croup** when air is forced through an obstructed larynx or trachea during inspiration. A snore is usually heard during sleep through an open mouth due to the vibration of the uvula and soft palate, can be soft or loud sound (Wilkins *et al.*, 2005). Sometimes it may be necessary to use a stethoscope placed on the chest to listen to sounds of inspiration. However, during auscultation, normal breath sounds should be bilateral and heard all over the lung zones (Bennett, 2003).

A nurse or a carer needs to observe the patient's chest wall or abdomen to observe the movement of breathing. When individuals are asked to breathe normally, they often think about their breathing and voluntarily change their respiratory rate and pattern. It is important that respiratory rate is assessed without the patient's awareness of the assessment. This precaution is not necessary with an unresponsive person (Baillie, 2005). You may also conduct this assessment by feeling the patient's abdomen to identify breathing rate or keep holding the wrist while observing the chest wall (Wilkins *et al.*, 2005). Respiratory distress can hinder speech where the patient is unable to complete full sentences or becomes monosyllabic, suffers from coughing or increased respiratory secretions (Bennett, 2003). However, respiratory monitoring must be completed to carry out prescribed interventions.

Activity 4.10

Reflect on an occasion when you have had an opportunity to assess respiration.
Recall if the patients were aware that you were counting their respirations. Do you think that this affected their rate or pattern of respiration? How long should you count respirations for?

While observing respiration, note the placement of the second hand on your fob watch and count each breath (in and out is one breath). Count the number of breaths over a minute to prevent error; never count for 10 or 15 s and multiply up to the minute. A holistic approach to management of respiratory difficulties includes physical, psychological, social and cognitive elements (Bennett, 2002); therefore, you will need to consider all aspects during an assessment.

For example

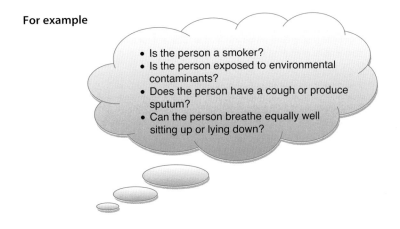

- Is the person a smoker?
- Is the person exposed to environmental contaminants?
- Does the person have a cough or produce sputum?
- Can the person breathe equally well sitting up or lying down?

During respiratory assessment, some patients may present with a cough. The cough reflex is stimulated by the entry of foreign body into the larynx, accumulation of secretions in the lower respiratory tract or inflammation causing irritation (Woodrow, 2002). If a patient experiences an episode of coughing, establish whether the cough is regular, duration of episode, whether it is associated with pain or produces any sound or sputum, or any trigger factors such as eating, drinking or smoking. Firstly, find out if it is productive or a non-productive cough. A non-productive cough is also called a dry cough. A productive cough expectorates sputum and during assessment observation of the character of sputum is helpful because it can indicate associated illness (Day, 2003). The characteristics of sputum include consistency (frothy, thick and watery), colour (white, black, pink, green yellow), quantity, frothy, mucoid, purulent appearance or blood stained and smell (see Table 4.4).

Table 4.4   The characteristics of sputum and associated conditions (*Source:* Adapted from Kennedy (2007, p. 44)).

Sputum	Associated conditions
Green, yellow thick and foul smelling	Infection
Blood stained	Tuberculosis, pulmonary embolism and lung cancer. Trauma
White, thick forthy sputum	Pulmonary oedema
Pink, frothy sputum	Heart failure
Brown, brick coloured	Tuberculosis and infection
Black	Tar in sputum seen in smokers

Activity 4.11

Practise how to record a respiratory rate on an observation chart (Table 4.5). Measure a volunteer's respiratory rate at rest in the first column. Then ask the volunteer to walk up and down a flight of stairs a couple of times and measure the respiratory rate; record this in the second column. After 10 min rest, monitor the respiratory rate and chart this in the third column. Mark with a cross.

    Now review the recording and note the differences at rest and exercise so that you can understand the importance of baseline readings.

Table 4.5   Observation chart: respiratory rate

Respiration per minute	Rest	Exercise	Rest

Communication

Patients who experience difficulty in respiration are usually distressed, restless, anxious and afraid (Jevon and Ewens, 2007), and sometimes fear that they may die. In extreme conditions, the patient can be pale, clammy and lethargic, and may present with a weak pulse or can be in shock or unconscious. Therefore, identifying these clinical symptoms (observe all vital signs) or understanding the patient's inability to verbalise effectively and recognising non-verbal cues (body language) are important to deliver prompt and optimal care. Furthermore, it is extremely important to constantly reassure the patient to allay anxiety and gain cooperation.

Your patient may be too weak or ill to talk/reply to your commands, so keep questions to a minimum.

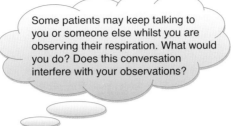

Some patients may keep talking to you or someone else whilst you are observing their respiration. What would you do? Does this conversation interfere with your observations?

Peak expiratory flow

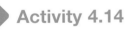 **Activity 4.12**

What is a peak flow meter?

Activity 4.13

When would you use a peak flow meter and why?

Activity 4.14

Where would you record a peak flow measurement?

Activity 4.15

What is the normal peak flow rate for an adult?

A peak flow meter is a small device that you blow into. It measures the amount of air (airflow) that can be blown out of the lungs; airflow is recorded in litres per minute (L/min). A peak flow meter is a hand-held instrument that measures an individual's ability to exhale (maximum size of expired breath). Usually, three measurements are taken and the highest of three is recorded (Woodrow, 2002). It measures the **peak expiratory flow rate** (PEFR) to determine the lung volume. This is performed after a full inspiration followed by a forced expiration through the meter (Miller et al., 2005); standard meters measure up to 1000 L/min (Jevon, 2007). A normal measurement can be influenced by a person's height, age and gender. Generally, males have a higher reading to females with an average adult measurement ranging from 400 to 600 L/min Baillie, 2005).

PEFR is commonly used for people with an acute exacerbation of asthma (Booker, 2007), when there is a degree of airway obstruction resulting in less air exhaled from the lungs per breath. Monitoring peak flow helps to determine whether asthma control is effective and especially useful in moderate to severe asthma. Further guidance on asthma management is available on the 'Asthma UK' website http://www.asthma.org.uk/.

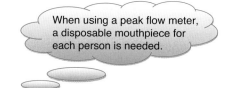

When using a peak flow meter, a disposable mouthpiece for each person is needed.

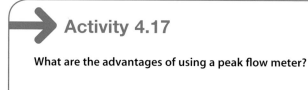

Activity 4.16

How often should the peak flow rate be measured?

Activity 4.17

What are the advantages of using a peak flow meter?

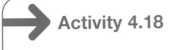

Activity 4.18

What are the disadvantages?

Each time you check your 'peak flow', you should do three blows, one after the other. The 'best of the three' is the reading to record. A common error associated with the recording of peal flow is that the people do not blow as hard as they can. Another error is that the people do not put their lips right around the mouthpiece to make sure that all the air they blow goes through the device.

Activity 4.19

Measure your own peak flow and record your readings in the table below. Usually, it is recorded at the bottom of the observation chart in clinical areas or others can self-monitor at home on self-designed charts or in a diary. You may find one in the skills laboratory or your clinical area.

	Peak flow measurement
Standing	
Sitting upright	
Lying flat	
After 5 min of brisk walking	

Compare your readings and discuss your experience of different positions during peak flow measurement. Correct technique on the use of the peak flow meter and upright position are vital to accurate measurement or else the patient can be mistreated (Booker, 2007). Always adhere to manufacturer's instruction on the procedure for use of peak flow meters. Peak flow is not measured in isolation, but the patient's health status and other observations are also considered. Although it is recommended to measure peak flow twice a day (morning and evening), it is advocated to monitor it before and 30 min after administration of bronchial dilators in acute cases to assess effectiveness of the medication (Moore, 2007). Accurate recording is important to maintain continuity of care and treatment.

Benefits of peak flow measurements in asthmatics

Peak flow measurements help to determine if asthma is controlled or to monitor respiratory status. The trends of recordings reveal deterioration or progress that instigates prompt evaluation of care. Therefore, medication can be changed to prevent an acute attack or preventive medication is considered if the patient's values are below 80% (Booker, 2007). Immediate medical attention is advised if the measurement is below 50% of the baseline.

Oxygen saturation rate — pulse oximetry

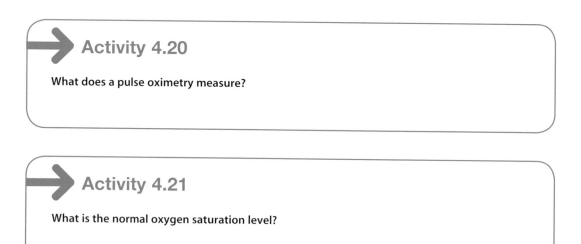

Activity 4.20

What does a pulse oximetry measure?

Activity 4.21

What is the normal oxygen saturation level?

This is non-invasive equipment that monitors the oxygen saturation of haemoglobin in arterial blood. There is a microprocessor with a probe attached to the patient that is easy to use and produces a quick reading. Examples of probes vary from a clip-on, sleeve, straps or tapes and are attached to fingers, toes, earlobes, or can be taped to the skin. There are different types of probes in various sizes available in practice and they can either be disposable or reusable (Chandler, 2000).

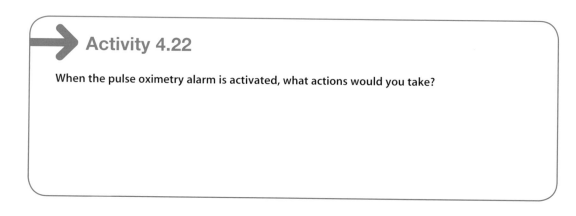

Activity 4.22

When the pulse oximetry alarm is activated, what actions would you take?

About 98% of oxygen is transported around the body by haemoglobin (Hb) in erythrocytes (red blood cells) (Baillie, 2005). The oxyhaemoglobin (HbO$_2$) rich in oxygen in the pulsating arterial vessels absorbs as much infrared light from the probe and the microprocessor produces the percentage of oxyhaemoglobin saturation. Therefore, a reliable reading depends on a tissue that has pulsatile flow of blood and a workable oximetry. A false reading can result if the light source has to pass through fat, bone, connective tissue, venous blood, dark nail vanish and poor peripheral circulation, disabling the photodetector (on the other side of the sensor) to absorb the red and infrared light (Baillie, 2005). Clinical conditions such as vasoconstriction, dysrhythmia and anaemia could influence accuracy of the pulse oximetry reading (Woodrow, 1999). However, oximetry can be used on acrylic nails that are not polished. It is pertinent to choose an appropriate probe to ensure the light-emitting diodes penetrate the vascular bed before reaching the photodetector.

Applying an oximetry on a finger of a blood pressure cuffed arm or attaching an ear probe over a pierced earlobe or damaged and poorly positioned probe would yield poor results (Neesam, 2000) and best results are obtained when the patient is at rest (Karnani *et al.*, 2005). Oximetry is commonly used with acutely ill patients, during investigations and surgery. Furthermore, those with respiratory and circulatory problems and those with **hypoxaemia** before **cyanosis** is visible should be monitored for at least 24 h when patients are on non-invasive ventilators (British Thoracic Society (BTS) 2002). The use of pulse oximetry has increasingly become routine in patient care and understanding how it works during monitoring is fundamental (Chandler, 2000) to nursing care. During a continuous reading, it is beneficial to check for skin damage due to pressure and is advisable to change the applicators on fingers and earlobes every 2–4 h (Docherty, 2002).

The greatest advantage of pulse oximetry is that it is a non-invasive piece of equipment that monitors oxygen saturations continuously eliminating frequent arterial blood gasses sampling. It also allows the healthcare professional to administer more or less oxygen as the condition dictates. However, pulse oximetry reading does not replace other vital signs observation and the patient's clinical manifestation must be taken into account (Walters, 2007). Any reading below 90% could indicate that the **pulse oximetry** equipment is faulty and unsafe for use (Kennedy, 2007). It is crucial to note that pulse oximetry cannot distinguish between different forms of saturated haemoglobin, distinctively carbohaemoglobin (COHb). Therefore, oximetry is not recommended for patients with carbon monoxide poisoning and tobacco smokers.

The normal **oxygen saturation** is 95–100% (Baillie, 2005). Any reading below 90% should be reported to a registered nurse or doctor immediately. However, the National Institute for Health and Clinical Excellence (NICE) accepts saturation observation between 90% and 93% only in patients with COPD (NICE, 2004). When the pulse oximetry alarm is activated, assess the patient first to see if patient is not in any distress, and then check the equipment. However, if the pulse oximetry reading remains low at rest or after exercise, it indicates gas exchange abnormalities and prompts further treatment (Karnani *et al.*, 2005), of which a nurse can usually prepare to administer oxygen (Chandler, 2000).

If you can access a pulse oximetry monitor, test your own reading.

Oxygen therapy

Oxygen therapy intervention is common in clinical practice. O_2 is a colourless and odourless gas that can be administrated in hospital, community and at home. Oxygen can be given short-term or for a long period of time and is delivered as continuous gaseous flow and measured in litres per minute. In many acute situations, it is the first drug (BMA *et al.*, 2001) to be given and is life saving. It should be prescribed (except in life threatening emergencies) at a recommended flow rate using variable oxygen administration devices (Bateman and Leach, 1998). The aim of oxygen therapy is to correct or reduce hypoxia. During hypoxia (lasting about 5 min), oxygenated blood can be decreased from 95% to 73% increasing respiratory rate from 18 to 24 breaths per minute (Yasuma and Hayano, 2008). The guideline from the British Thoracic Society (BTS) on emergency use of oxygen in adults is currently available from www.brit-thoracic.org.uk.

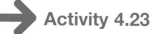

Activity 4.23

Why is oxygen therapy necessary? Who needs it?

In practice, you may have encountered situations when oxygen therapy is administered. It is commonly used during cardiac or respiratory arrest and shock, after general anaesthetics, heart attack, chest and truncal injuries and respiratory distress (asthma, COPD, bronchitis, and cystic fibrosis). It is also important to document the start and finish date of the treatment, time of oxygen therapy, including concentration of oxygen delivered.

Activity 4.24

What is hypoxia?

Activity 4.25

List the signs and symptoms of hypoxia.

Activity 4.26

Look around in your clinical area or skills laboratory for various types of oxygen apparatus and delivery devices. Identify the oxygen flow meter, oxygen gauge, appropriate adaptors for different size tubing and oxygen masks.

Methods of delivery of oxygen therapy

- There are various oxygen concentrations measured in percentages such as 24%, 28%, 35%, 40%, 60% and 100%.
- Flow meters deliver oxygen in litres per minute and the flow corresponds to desired oxygen concentration and respective devices used such as mask, venturi mask, nasal cannula and non-breathing mask (all single-use disposables).
- All equipment used must be disposed as per trust policy.

Oxygen masks can be divided into two groups.

1. Low flow rate masks (nasal cannula, simple face masks and masks with a reservoir bag) deliver oxygen at less than the peak inspiratory flow rate. They therefore deliver a variable concentration of oxygen, depending on how the patients are breathing.
2. High flow rate masks (sometimes called Venturi masks) deliver oxygen at a rate above the peak inspiratory flow rate, which is why they are noisier. They deliver fixed concentrations of oxygen. Figure 4.3 is an example of an oxygen mask on a patients face.

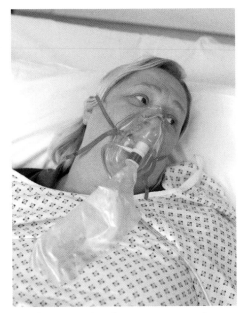

Figure 4.3   An example of an oxygen mask on a patient's face

Mask selection

- Correct mask and flow rate is vital during oxygen delivery based on oxygen concentration required and patient's ability to be complacent.
- Concentration of oxygen is decided depending on patient's presenting symptoms, oximetry reading or blood gas analysis.

Simple oxygen mask

Simple face masks and masks with a reservoir bag are used where higher concentrations of oxygen are required and controlled oxygen is not necessary, for example severe asthma, acute left ventricular failure, pneumonia, trauma or severe sepsis. Masks should always be set to a minimum of 5 L/min because significant re-breathing of CO_2 can occur when exhaled air is not adequately flushed from the mask; this is recommended to deliver approximately 35%–70% oxygen concentration (Oh and Seo, 2003). You must be cautious when the flow rate is below 4 L/min due to accumulation of expired carbon dioxide within the mask and risk of re-breathing exhaled carbon dioxide (Hickey, 2007).

Venturi mask

A Venturi mask is for controlled treatment with oxygen required in people with chronic respiratory failure, for example COPD. This is supplied with different coloured fittings indicating specific oxygen concentrations with recommended flow rates. The fittings include entry of ambient air to be diluted with oxygen flow before it reaches the patient. You will be expected to administer the prescribed concentration of oxygen using the appropriate fitting and regulate the required flow rate. Approximately 24%–60% of oxygen concentration could be delivered (Jevon and Ewens, 2001).

Nasal cannula

These are recommended for patients with normal vital signs, for example post-operative, slightly low oxygen saturations, long-term treatment with oxygen at home. Nasal prongs are a thin tube with two small nozzles that protrude directly into the patient's nostrils. It is estimated to deliver approximately 2–4 L/min of 25%–40% oxygen concentration (Bourke, 2003). Vines *et al.* (2000) commend that it is cheap and well tolerated by patients. However, nasal mucosa dryness can result with flow rate of more than 4 L/min is used. Traditionally, if you wanted to administer supplemental oxygen to a patient at a flow rate greater than 6 L/min, you could not use a nasal cannula; you would have to use a mask delivery system instead. However, there are two high-flow nasal cannula systems now available which may provide an option for various patients, including those who need high-flow oxygen but cannot tolerate a mask (Pruitt 2007).

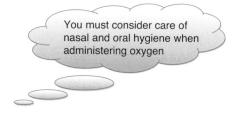

You must consider care of nasal and oral hygiene when administering oxygen

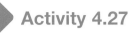 Activity 4.27

In your skills laboratory, under supervision, practise administering oxygen using a nasal cannula on a mannequin and then try using the simple oxygen mask. Note the differences between the two different devices used. Consider how to loosen or tighten the nasal cannula.

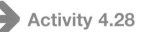 Activity 4.28

What are the advantages and disadvantages of giving oxygen via nasal cannula?

Humidified oxygen is the administration of oxygen using a humidifier to prevent dryness of the mouth and nostrils. Non-humidified oxygen dries the mouth and nostrils resulting in sticky chest secretions making it difficult to expectorate (Baillie, 2005). Frequent mouthwashes, oral care and increased fluid intake help to maintain moist upper respiratory environment. However, you must not use petroleum jelly, which is potentially flammable to prevent burns (Porter-Jones, 2002). Humidification is necessary when oxygen is delivered for long period (more than 12 h) or high oxygen concentration (more than 35%) and if delivered via tracheostomy or endotracheal tube (Baillie, 2005).

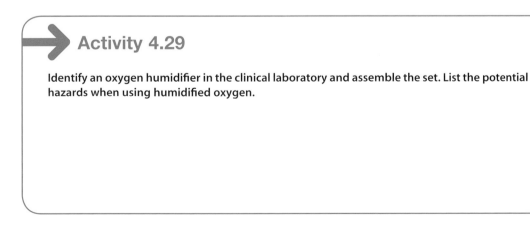 Activity 4.29

Identify an oxygen humidifier in the clinical laboratory and assemble the set. List the potential hazards when using humidified oxygen.

Table 4.6   Differences in cold and hot water oxygen humidifiers

Cold water system oxygen	Heated water system oxygen
Bubbles through water at room temperature	Bubbles across a heated reservoir of water
Usually used for short-term treatment	This is more efficient than cold water system
Disadvantage	**Disadvantages**
May cause reflex bronchoconstriction	1. Potential over-heating of mucous membrane or burning 2. Oxygen flow can be impeded due to excessive condensation in the tubing
Cheap and user friendly	More expensive than cold water system

Sterile water is used and changed daily to minimise bacterial contamination as a moist environment promotes multiplication of bacteria. Humidified oxygen can be provided via cold water or heated water systems (adhere to manufacturer's recommendation). Refer to Table 4.6 for the differences in cold and hot water oxygen humidifiers.

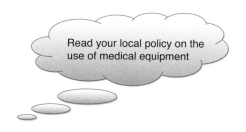

Read your local policy on the use of medical equipment

However, the heated water system oxygen humidifiers are more popular in acute care settings than cold water system oxygen, may be due to severity of patient's illness.

Equipment

- Oxygen delivery system, appropriate mask, humidification equipment.
- In hospitals, oxygen is supplied either via cylinders (black with white shoulders) or via wall-mounted oxygen pipes (yellow).
- Oxygen cylinders are portable, can be of different sizes/volumes and can be heavy. They must be well secured during transport, usage and storage to prevent damage and injury to users and those helping to assemble the apparatus, visitors and others. Replacements must be readily available.

- A pressure regulator is used to control the high pressure of oxygen delivered from a cylinder to a low pressure controllable by the flow meter.
- A flow meter is used to control and indicate the flow of oxygen (flow range is 0–15 L/min). This can be regulated to deliver low to high flow but the dial must be checked periodically to ensure the cylinder is not empty.

Risks of oxygen treatment

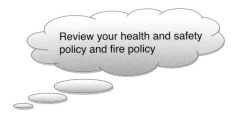

Review your health and safety policy and fire policy

Fire hazards

Oxygen supports combustion and using it together with other inflammable items such as cigarettes can start a fire. Therefore, strictly no smoking and avoid gadgets or toys that can cause sparks.

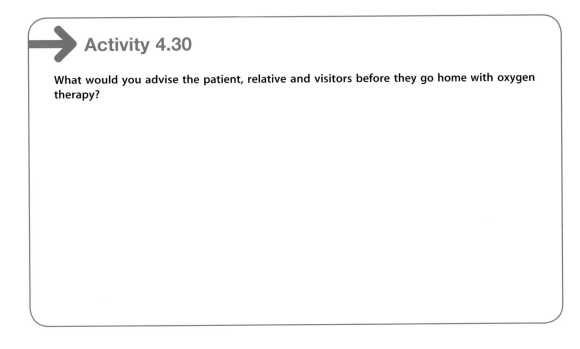

Activity 4.30

What would you advise the patient, relative and visitors before they go home with oxygen therapy?

Carbon dioxide retainers

Some patients with chronic respiratory disease such as COPD and cystic fibrosis normally have a high level of carbon dioxide in their blood and are referred to as CO_2 retainers. These patient's chemoreceptors no longer stimulate respiration; therefore, lack of oxygen stimulates breathing (in normal people, an increase in CO_2 stimulates respiration). Hence, care must be taken when oxygen is delivered to patients with respiratory diseases; only 24%–28% of oxygen is normally prescribed (Baillie, 2005). When a high percentage of oxygen is given to some patients with respiratory disease, they can develop carbon dioxide narcosis leading to coma (Porter-Jones, 2002).

The British Thoracic Society (British Thoracic Society, 2006) statistics remain alarming as respiratory disease kills 1:4 (2001) and 1:5 (2006) people in the UK and costs the National Health Service over £6 billion. This report emphasises the pivotal focus on health promotion and this is the integral part of our role as a nurse to encourage smoking cessation, healthy life-style, exercise and compliance to drug therapy, if any prescribed (French, 2003; Whyte, 2004). The benefits of exercise are clearly evident with pulmonary rehabilitation programmes, mainly exercise, including different activities and body posture in daily life has improved functional capacity (Pitta et al., 2008).

Activity 4.31

Reflect on your placement experience when you cared for patients with breathing difficulty. Write in sentences what happened, how you felt and what would you do differently (if anything) next time when you monitor and assess respiration.

What happened?

How did it make you feel?

What would you do differently (if anything) next time?

Case Studies: Consider the case studies below and discuss some of the issues with your mentor or supervisor at work.

Case study 4.1

Mr Smith is in a medical ward with chronic bronchitis. He is breathless and has a productive cough. He had been left in the day room to watch TV with a portable oxygen cylinder. Now he wants to go back to bed to rest and has asked for your help. How would you assist Mr Smith to his bed? Consider his breathlessness, oxygen cylinder and a box of tissue where he expectorates his sputum. Would you ask for another nurse to help you? How would you transfer Mr Smith from day room to his bedside?

Case study 4.2

Upon reaching Mr Smith's bedside, his bed is flat and the nearest wall-mounted oxygen supply is being used by another patient. What would you do? After transferring the patient safely to bed and making him comfortable in an upright position, you notice the oxygen supply in the cylinder is getting low. How would you manage this situation? *Consider reporting to your mentor and prepare another oxygen cylinder as standby or find out if the other patient has any other wall-mounted oxygen port nearer to him.*

Case study 4.3

During the change of oxygen cylinder, Mr Smith becomes very anxious and has difficulty in breathing with an occasional wheeze. How would you allay Mr Smith's anxiety and what other actions would you consider? Effective listening and good communication skills are essential in reassuring Mr Smith to minimise anxiety induced breathlessness. Perform respiratory assessment besides pulse and blood pressure recording and document them accurately in the clinical chart. Report to staff immediately and continue observation of respiration. Sometimes medication is administered to relief wheeze, and if condition deteriorates, the medical team may need to be summoned.

Case study 4.4

If Mr Smith's condition deteriorates, a peak flow meter reading may be requested. Consider Mr Smith's difficulties in using the peak flow meter. He might be sitting forward a little and not able to fully expand his lungs to maximum capacity. Compare the current reading with the previous reading. Discuss the peak flow trend with your mentor to determine any changes in treatment.

Chapter summary

Respiratory care involves observation of the patient's chest wall movements to recognise rate, pattern and depth to enable you to implement appropriate care for the patient. It is important to monitor and report to the nurse in charge when measurements deviate from the normal range or when patient's condition deteriorates.

There is a variety of medical equipment available to enhance the care being delivered but complete reliance on modern technology should be avoided (Walters, 2007) and the patient must be assessed first, especially, when the medical devices activate an alarm. However, respiratory monitoring and assessment involves observation of general appearance, effectiveness of breathing, speech, use of a peak flow meter, pulse oximetry, oxygen therapy and health promotion (French, 2003). The use of medical devices is increasingly popular and user friendly (Brown *et al.*, 2006); nevertheless, it is still the individual nurses' responsibility to ensure its safety and appropriateness (Walters, 2007). However, initial assessment can be undertaken without the aid of medical devices (Woodrow, 2002).

Nurses have become central to the delivery of respiratory care in both primary and secondary settings; though this can be timely and inappropriately performed at times. However, failure to provide necessary and appropriate respiratory care can adversely affect patient outcome. Respiratory care is constantly changing, so try to be aware of what is current and new, so that you can help the patient to receive safe and appropriate care.

Answers to Activities

Activity 4.1 Your thoughts on witnessing someone with respiratory difficulties

These are your thoughts and personal to you. However, fear and anxiety can be overcome by knowledge and experience. Practice makes perfect and applying underpinning knowledge strengthens confidence and develops competence.

Activity 4.2 Key terms

Term	Definition
Tachypnoea	Rapid breathing that exceeds normal rate (>18 breaths per minute)
Bradypnoea	Slow rate of breathing, lower than normal rate (<12 breaths per minute)
Apnoea	Absence of breathing
Eupnoea	Normal, unlaboured breathing (between 10 and 17 breaths per minute)
Cheyne–Stokes	Abnormal breathing with alternating periods of shallow and deep breathing, also with periods of apnoea
Stridor	A harsh, shrill, grating or cracking sound; usually with a partial block during inspiration
Respiration	Includes inspiration and expiration
Oxygen saturation	Peripheral measurement of amount of oxygen in the blood
Peak flow	Measurement of forced expired air in litres per minute after a forced inspiration (changes in breathing capacity)

Activity 4.3

When would you monitor a patient's respiratory rate?

- On arrival or before admission of a patient
- Before the start of procedure or pre-operatively to act as baseline
- When patient's condition deteriorates or improves
- Post surgery, during treatment (e.g. on morphine infusion)
- Monitor response to treatment or medication.

Activity 4.4

Using an anatomy and physiology textbook, label the diagram in Figure 4.2, then write down the function of each section of the respiratory system.

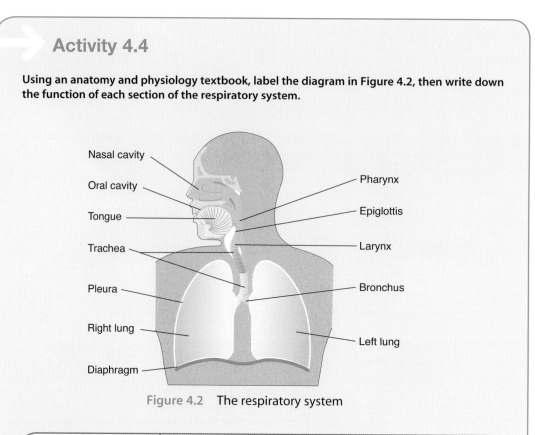

Nasal cavity

Oral cavity

Tongue

Trachea

Pleura

Right lung

Diaphragm

Pharynx

Epiglottis

Larynx

Bronchus

Left lung

Figure 4.2   The respiratory system

Key word	Function
Nostril	
Mouth	
Pharynx	
Epiglottis	
Larynx	
Trachea	
Bronchus	
Alveoli	
Diaphragm	

Please refer to any anatomy and physiology textbook and review the respiratory system and you will be able to find all answers for the table.

Activity 4.5

What is the normal respiratory rate for an adult?

Respiratory pattern is an effortless rhythm of breathing, with usually equal inspiration and expiration ratio. The average rate for an adult is between 12 and 18 breaths per minute.

Activity 4.6

Describe what you understand by respiratory pattern.

Respiratory pattern is an effortless rhythm of breathing, with usually equal inspiration and expiration ratio.

Activity 4.7

Outline the factors that are important when assessing respiratory depth.

The important factors when assessing respiratory depth are as follows:

- Recognise duration of inspiration and expiration phases, usually directly proportional to each other
- Respiratory depth can be shallow or deep/rapid or slow and the volume of air in each inspiration and expiration differs accordingly
- Observe or feel chest movement or listen to breath sounds
- Observe for equal expansion of both sides of the chest

Nursing assessment
- Observation of general appearance
- Breathing patterns (as above)
- Abnormal chest movement
- Signs of laboured breathing
- Skin colour
- Breath odour
- Emotional state of the person

Activity 4.8

During a respiratory assessment of a patient, you notice that the patient is tachypnoeic and you wonder why there is an increase in his or her respiratory rate.

List below some factors that could cause tachypnoea.

- Stress
- Fear
- Exercise
- Fever
- Anxiety
- Pain
- Respiratory diseases (e.g. atelectasis)

Activity 4.9

Using an anatomy and physiology textbook, list below the accessory muscles of respiration.

Accessory muscle of respiration:

- Sternocleidomastoid — passes obliquely across the side of the neck
- Scalenus — muscles at the side of the neck
- Trapezius — muscles spanning from the neck
- Pectoral muscles — upper front of the chest wall

Activity 4.10

Reflect on an occasion when you have had an opportunity to assess respiration.
    Recall if the patients were aware that you were counting their respirations. Do you think that this affected their rate or pattern of respiration? How long should you count respirations for?

These are your thoughts and personal to you. However, fear and anxiety can be overcome by knowledge and experience. The opportunity to assess respiration can be your first experience or any situation that was challenging where the patient was unwell or dyspnoeic.

- Did you observe respiration by watching the chest wall or did you feel by placing your hand on patient's chest?
- Did you count the respiratory rate for one full minute and record it immediately?
- Could you recognise the pattern/rhythm and depth and able to identify Cheyne–Stoke respiration or hyperventilation?
- If there were previous measurements to compare, what did the trend of respiratory recording imply?

Nursing assessment

- Observation of general appearance
- Breathing patterns (as above)
- Abnormal chest movement
- Signs of laboured breathing
- Skin colour
- Breath odour
- Emotional state of the person

Activity 4.11

Practise how to record a respiratory rate on an observation chart (Table 4.5). Measure a volunteer's respiratory rate at rest in the first column. Then ask the volunteer to walk up and down a flight of stairs a couple of times and measure the respiratory rate; record this in the second column. After 10 min rest, monitor the respiratory rate and chart this in the third column. Mark with a cross.

Activity 4.11 (Continued)

Now review the recording and note the differences at rest and exercise so that you can understand the importance of baseline readings.

These are your volunteer's measurements. This opportunity to assess your volunteer can take place at your accommodation, in clinical laboratory or practice area. This exercise can be enjoyable and fun.

- Did you observe respiration by watching the chest wall or did you feel by placing your hand on your volunteer's chest?
- Did you count the respiratory rate for one full minute?
- Did you remember the measurement when recording it?
- Could you recognise the pattern/rhythm and depth?
- What did the respiratory trend in your chart demonstrate?
- Was your volunteer's respiration return to resting values after exercise?

Table 4.5   Observation chart: respiratory rate

	Rest	Exercise	Rest
Respiration per minute			

Activity 4.12

What is a peak flow meter?

Peak flow meter is an instrument that measures the maximum size of expired breath.

Activity 4.13

When would you use a peak flow meter and why?

Usually used by asthmatic patients or when someone has shortness of breath. This is used to establish physiological measurements of the lung capacity to help to decide appropriate treatment. Normally pre- and post-treatment (inhalers) readings are recorded (Miller *et al.*, 2005).

Activity 4.14

Where would you record a peak flow measurement?

It is good practice to record readings immediately after taking them in order not to forget. Please refer to local practice where to document reading, either in nursing notes with date and time or clinical charts or observation charts.

Activity 4.15

What is the normal peak flow rate for an adult?

Normal values can vary based on a person's age, sex and size.
It is difficult to say exactly what a person's best peak flow should be.
For example you can expect:

- 25-year-old man, who is 6 feet 1 inch (185 cm or 1.85 m) tall, to have an average peak flow of 627 L/min.
- 40-year-old woman, who is 5 feet 2 inches (157 cm or 1.57 m) tall, to have an average peak flow of 427 L/min.

However, a person's peak flow could be less than this and still be completely normal (Partridge, 2008).

Activity 4.16

How often should the peak flow rate be measured?

Peak flow measurements are most useful when a person is able to take and compare peak flow measurements on a day-to-day basis.

- Commonly used by asthmatic patients
- Generally twice a day (morning and evening)
- During acute illness – before and 30 min after administration of bronchodilators
- During acute illness symptoms such as increased cough, shortness of breath, wheezing alters the recording from normal range demonstrating requirement for treatment
- The differences between each reading will show whether asthma is being properly controlled

Activity 4.17

What are the advantages of using a peak flow meter?

- Measurement done within 1–2 min
- Inexpensive
- Simple and safe

Activity 4.18

What are the disadvantages?

- It is dependent on effort from the patient
- Insensitive to obstruction of smaller airways
- Much less accurate than spirometers
- Reading is difficult to achieve during hypothermia/nail varnish/carbon monoxide poisoning

Activity 4.19

Measure your own peak flow and record your readings in the table below. Usually, it is recorded at the bottom of the observation chart in clinical areas or others can self-monitor at home on self-designed charts or in a diary. You may find one in the skills laboratory or your clinical area.

	Peak flow measurement
Standing	
Sitting upright	
Lying flat	
After 5 min of brisk walking	

Activity 4.20

What does a pulse oximetry measure?

It measures oxygen saturation.

Activity 4.21

What is the normal oxygen saturation level?

The normal oxygen saturation level is 95–100%.

Activity 4.22

When the pulse oximetry alarm is activated, what actions would you take?

● Stop the alarm that may be distressing to patient and to reduce noise pollution.
● Immediately assess patient's condition before checking whether the equipment is faulty.
● If patient condition has deteriorated, alert the medical team.
● If the patient's condition remains stable then look for any fault in the oximetry; commonly, the sensor applicator (finger or ear clip) slips off.
● Re-attach the used sensor applicators or replace with another to continue care.

Activity 4.23

Why is oxygen therapy necessary? Who needs it?

Oxygen therapy is commenced to boost the oxygen saturation level and alleviate clinical symptoms such as hypoxia, shortness of breath, general anaesthesia, life threatening situation, anaphylaxis, and so on.

Activity 4.24

What is hypoxia?

Hypoxia is the deficiency of oxygen in the tissues.

Activity 4.25

List the signs and symptoms of hypoxia.

● Rapid breathing
● Breathing that is distressed or gasping
● Difficulty in speaking
● Grey-blue skin (cyanosis)
● Anxiety
● Restlessness
● Headache
● Nausea and possible vomiting
● Cessation of breathing if hypoxia is not quickly reversed

(First Aid Manual, 2006).

Activity 4.26

Look around in your clinical area or skills laboratory for various types of oxygen apparatus and delivery devices. Identify the oxygen flow meter, oxygen gauge, appropriate adaptors for different size tubing and oxygen masks.

This task can be carried out in the clinical laboratory or practice placement area; identify all the required equipment and assemble apparatus under supervision. If unsure, ask your supervisor or mentor or refer to clinical poster and book. Always adhere to manufacturer's recommendation. This is a useful exercise where you can assemble the equipment without being rushed for clinical need and errors can be rectified.

Activity 4.27

In your skills laboratory, under supervision, practise administering oxygen using a nasal cannula on a mannequin and then try using the simple oxygen mask. Note the differences between the two different devices used. Consider how to loosen or tighten the nasal cannula.

This exercise helps you enhance the delivery of oxygen therapy and how to fit a face mask or nasal cannula over a patient's face. Identify which straps to pull in order to secure and snug fit the mask or nasal cannula to avoid pressure development. Should you first turn on the prescribed oxygen before putting the face mask or nasal cannula or put on the mask/cannula and then turn on the oxygen? Turn on oxygen before applying the mask or cannula over the patient's face to avoid sudden gush of air and it is advisable to prime the tubing before oxygen administration.

Activity 4.28

What are the advantages and disadvantages of giving oxygen via nasal cannula?

Advantages of nasal cannula:

- Cheap and well tolerated by patient
- Oxygen is administered directly into the nostril avoiding accumulation of expired air in front of nose and mouth (may happen when a face mask is used)
- Patient can eat, drink and talk more easily without disruption of oxygen administration

Disadvantages of nasal cannula:

- Only 25%–40% oxygen concentration is recommended (2–6 L/min)
- May not deliver accurate or actual oxygen level
- Dries nasal mucosa
- Risk of pressure sore development behind ears

Activity 4.29

Identify an oxygen humidifier in the clinical laboratory and assemble the set. List the potential hazards when using humidified oxygen.

This task can be carried out in the clinical laboratory or practice placement area. Identify all the required equipment and assemble apparatus under supervision. If unsure, ask your supervisor or mentor or refer to clinical poster and book. Always adhere to manufacturer's recommendation. This is a useful exercise where you can assemble the equipment unhurriedly away from clinical area.

Potential hazards of using humidified oxygen:

● Apply all oxygen therapy precautions.
● Dehydration: Dryness of mouth and nostrils leading to sticky chest secretions.
● Potentially flammable: Avoid petroleum jelly or alcohol-based spray.
● Infection: Water used must be sterile, changed daily, re-filled as the water level drops due evaporation.

Activity 4.30

What would you advise the patient, relative and visitors before they go home with oxygen therapy?

Patient, relative and visitors both in hospital and during home oxygen therapy must be informed of the fire hazard. Please attend fire lectures to understand the 'fire triangle' (oxygen, fuel and heat – all three must be present to start a fire). Oxygen supports combustion and the following must be reinforced (Baillie, 2005):

● No smoking sign
● No toys or devices that can spark
● Explain the risk of smoking during oxygen therapy (perfume, aftershave, and alcohol-based sprays).
● Knowledge of fire procedure and equipment
● Home-use oxygen cylinders must be stored away from gas fires, naked flames and hot radiators.

Activity 4.31

Reflect on your placement experience when you cared for patients with breathing difficulty. Write in sentences what happened, how you felt and what would you do differently (if anything) next time when you monitor and assess respiration.

This is your personal experience of caring for a patient with breathing difficulty. Reflect your own personal feelings in relation to your learning needs. You may have more than one learning need; hence, you could use the same subheadings to address the issues.

What happened?

● Describe the scenario briefly relating to your learning need.

Activity 4.31 (Continued)

How did it make you feel?

- Did you feel good or bad about it?
- What was good or bad about the situation?
- Did you have adequate underpinning knowledge to carry out the care?
- If you had previous experience of similar situation, was it useful this time?

What would you do differently (if anything) next time?

- Has this personal experience prepared you to do further reading and gained more practice under supervision?

This is only a guide. Please address the subheadings to meet your own learning needs.

References

Ahern, J. and Phipot, P. (2002) Assessing acutely ill patient on general wards. *Nursing Standard* **16** (47), 57–54.

Baillie, L. (2005) *Developing Practical Skills*, 2nd edn (London: Hodder Arnold).

Bateman, N. and Leach, R. (1998) ABC of oxygen: acute oxygen therapy. *British Medical Journal* **317**, 798–801.

Benner, P. (1984) *From Novice to Expert: Excellence and Power in Clinical Nursing Practice* (California: Addison Wesley).

Bennett, C. (2002) Respiratory care. In *Key Nursing Skills*, B. Workman and C. Bennett, eds (London: Whurr).

Bennett, C. (2003) Nursing the breathless patient. *Nursing Standard* **17** (17), 45–51.

Booker, R. (2007) Peak expiratory low measurement. *Nursing Standard* **21** (39), 42–43.

Bozkurt, B. and Mann, D. (2003) Shortness of breath. *Journal of the American Heart Association* **108**, e11–e13.

British Medical Association, Resuscitation Council UK and Royal College of Nursing (2001) *Decisions Relating to Cardiopulmonary Resuscitation: A Joint Statement* (London: BMA).

British Thoracic Society (BTS) (2002) Standards of care committee non invasive ventilation in acute respiratory failure. *Thorax* **57**, 192–211.

British Thoracic Society (2006) *The Burden of Lung Disease, A Statistics Report* (London: Department of Health).

Brown, R., DiMarco, A., Hoit, J. and Garshick, E. (2006) Respiratory dysfunction and management in spinal cord injury. *Respiratory Care* **51** (8), 853–870.

Bourke, S. (2003) *Respiratory Medicine*, 6th edn (Oxford: Blackwell).

Casey, G. (2001) Oxygen transport and the use of pulse oximetry. *Nursing Standard* **15** (47), 46–53.

Chandler, T. (2000) Oxygen saturation monitoring. *Paediatric Nursing* **12** (8), 37–42.

Chellel, A., Fraser, J. and Fender, V. (2002) Nursing observation on ward patients at risk of critical illness. *Nursing Times* **98** (46), 36–39.

Day, M. (2003) A rapid access and early discharge service for people with COPD. *Nursing Times* **99** (20), 44–45, supplement.

Docherty, B. (2002) Cardiorespiratory physical assessment for the acutely ill. *British Journal of Nursing* **11** (11), 750–758.

DoH (2001) *The Essence of Care: Patient-Focused Benchmarking for Health Care Practitioners* (London: Department of Health).

First Aid Manual (2006) *Step by Step Guide for Everyone. St.John Ambulance, St Andrew's Ambulance Association* (London: British Red Cross).

French, J. (2003) Developing effective services for people with COPD. *Nursing Times* **99** (20), 48, supplement.

Glasper, E., McEwing, G. and Richardson, J. (2007) *Oxford Handbook of Children's & Yound People's Nursing* (Oxford: Oxford University Press).

Hickey, S. (2007) An audit of oxygen therapy on a respiratory ward. *British Journal of Nursing* **16** (18), 32–36.

Jevon, P. (2007) Respiratory procedures. *Nursing Times* **103** (33), 26–27.

Jevon, P. and Ewens, B. (2001) Assessment of a breathless patient. *Nursing Standard* **15** (16), 48–53.

Jevon, P. and Ewens, B. (2007) *Monitoring the Critically Ill Patient*, 2nd edn (Oxford: Blackwell Science).

Karnani, N., Reisfield, G. and Wilson, G. (2005) Evaluation of chronic dyspnoea. *American Family Physician* **71** (8), 1465–1538.

Kennedy, S. (2007) Detecting changes in the respiratory status of ward patients. *Nursing Standard* **21** (49), 42–46.

Kenward, G. (2001) Time to put the 'R' back to TPR. *Nursing Times* **97** (40), 32–33.

Miller, M., Hankinson, J., Brusasco, V., Burgos, F., Casaburi, R., Coates, A., *et al.* (2005) ATS/ERS Task Force: standardisation of spirometry. *European Respiratory Journal* **26** (2), 319–338.

Moore, T. (2007) Respiratory assessment in adults. *Nursing Standard* **21** (49), 48–56.

National Institute of Health and Clinical Excellence (2004) *Chronic Obstructive Pulmonary Disease. Management of Chronic Obstructive Pulmonary Disease in Adults in Primary and Secondary Care. Clinical Guidelines 12* (London: NICE).

Neesam, N. (2000) Pulse oximetry in practice. *Nursing Standard* **14** (30), 55.

NMC (2008) *The Code: Standards of Conduct, Performance and Ethics for Nurse and Midwives* (London: Nursing and Midwifery Council), p. 10.

Oh H and Seo W (2003) A meta-analysis of the effects of various interventions in preventing endotracheal suction-induced hypoxemia. *Journal of Clinical Nursing* **12**, 912–924.

Partridge, M. (2008) National Asthma Campaign. http://www.netdoctor.co.uk/diseases/facts/asthmapeakflowmeter.htm (accessed 29 April 2008).

Pitta, F., Troosters, T., Probst, V., Langer, D., Decramer, M. and Gosselink, R. (2008) Are patients with COPD more active after pulmonary rehabilitation? *Chest*. http//chestjournal.org/cgi/content/abstract/chest.07-2655v1 (accessed 25 April 2008).

Porter-Jones, G. (2002) Short-term oxygen therapy. *Nursing Times* **98** (40), 53–56.

Pruitt, B. (2007) Latest advances in critical care. *Critical Care* **37** (7), 56–59.

Vines, D., Shelledy, D. and Peters, J. (2000) Current respiratory care, Part 1; Oxygen therapy, oximetry, bronchial hygiene. *Journal of Critical Illness* **15**, 507–505.

Walters, T. (2007) Pulse oximetry knowledge and its effects on clinical practice. *British Journal of Nursing* **16** (21), 332–340.

Wilkins, R., Sheldon, R. and Krider, S. (2005) *Clinical Assessment in Respiratory Care*, 5th edn (Missouri: Elsevier Mosby).

Whyte, A. (2004) Expanding respiratory care. *Nursing Times* **100** (9), 20–29.

Woodrow, P. (1999) Pulse oximetry. *Nursing Standard* **13** (42), 42–46.

Woodrow, P. (2002) Assessing respiratory function in older people. *Nursing Older People* **14** (3), 27–28.

Yasuma, F. and Hayano, J. (2008) Respiratory sinus arrhythmia: why does the heartbeat synchronise with respiratory rhythm? *Chest* **125** (2), 683–690.

Further reading

Baillie, J. (2008) Simple, easily memorised 'rules of thumb' for the rapid assessment of physiological compensation for respiratory acid–base disorders. *Thorax* **63**, 289–290.

Booker, E. (2008) Respiratory assessment. *Nursing Standard* **22** (21), 59.

Finch, J. and Berrisford, M. (2001) *Greater Manchester Multi Professional Critical Care – Respiratory 1 Workbook*, 3rd edn (Greater Manchester Strategic Health Authority: NHS).

Kennedy, S. (2006) Assessment of a patient with an acute exacerbation of Asthma. *Nursing Standard* **21** (4), 35–38.

Richardson, M. (2003) Physiology for practice: the mechanisms controlling respiration. *Nursing Times* **99** (48), 48–50.

Montague, S., Watson, R. and Herbert, R. (2005) *Physiology for Nursing Practice*, 5th edn (London: Bailliere Tindall).

Watson, D. (2006) The impact of accurate patient assessment on quality care. *Nursing Times* **100** (34), 34–35.

Weller, B. (2005) *Bailliere's Nurses Dictionary*, 24th edn (London: Bailliere Tindall).

Williams, J. (201) Development of a self reported chronic respiratory questionnaire (CRQ-SR). *Thorax* **56**, 954–959.

Useful websites

Asthma UK: www.asthma.org.uk

British Lung Foundation: www.britishlungfoundation.com

British Thoracic Society: www.brit-thoracic.org.uk

Oxygen Therapy: www.wikipedia.org/wiki/Oxygen_therapy

http://images.main.uab.edu/healthsys/ei_0372.gif

www.goldcopd.com

5 Principles of nutritional care

THOMAS BEARY

→ **Aims**

The aim of this chapter is to introduce you to the key principles of nutritional care and provide an overview of the factors that determines patient's ability to eat and drink.

→ **Learning objectives**

On completion of this chapter, you will learn to:
- Understand the principles of eating and drinking
- Outline the importance of the assessment of eating and drinking needs and their importance within care delivery
- Understand the significance of the different nutrients which must be obtained from food
- Appreciate the meaning of assessment of needs to determine nutritional status
- Identify the practicalities of meeting nutritional needs

Introduction

This chapter will explore the importance of eating and drinking in everyday life whilst considering the knowledge and skills which are essential in acknowledging the significance of such tasks. A working knowledge of the issues associated with nutritional needs is essential for all nurses to ensure that appropriate care is delivered to the patients in our care. It will also explore the importance of nutritional care at times of ill health as well as highlighting the value of intervention at this crucial time. The completion of activities will be central to this chapter since such activities will allow you to identify the crucial issues associated with the activities of eating and drinking, especially in the light of essential nursing care delivery. Some case studies will be utilised which may or may not require discussion or reflection. However, these case studies will highlight pertinent issues and such case studies are taken from real-life situations. All names have been changed to protect confidentiality (Nursing and Midwifery Council, 2008). In light of this, please read the first case study.

Activity 5.1 Key terms

Before discussing the issues associated with eating and drinking, it is essential to understand key terms. Use a dictionary and other literature to find a definition for each of the following key terms. Alternatively, you can discuss the following terms with other healthcare professionals such as registered nurses, doctors and dieticians.

Term	Definition
Nutrition	
Malnourishment	
Kilocalorie	
Obesity	
Diet	
Mastication	
Digestion	
Absorption	
Metabolism	
Dehydration	
Intestine	
Electrolyte	

Activity 5.1 (*Continued*)

Peristalsis	
Chyme	
Stomach	
Nitrogen	
Magnesium	
Calcium	
Potassium	
Assessment	
Carnivorous	
Omnivorous	
Vegetarian	
Vegan	
Halal	
Kosher	
Orthodox	
Diffusion	
Osmosis	
Intracellular	
Extracellular	
Oedema	
Diuretic	
Homeostasis	

According to McFerran and Martin (2003), nutrition is the study of food in relation to the physiological processes that depend on its absorption by the body. Say (2005a) suggests that nutrition involves a specific course of action by which cells receive and use food material or nutrients to support and maintain metabolism in all parts of the body. Maintaining a sufficient intake of food and fluids is required for our very existence but, more importantly, it is essential for our fitness and welfare both in sickness and in health and for the prevention of unintentional weight loss in the form of malnutrition (Smith, 2008). Consequently, Heath (1995) suggests that there may be many health problems which could be directly linked to nutrition. Heath (1995) also points out that good nutrition does not always lead to good health, but good health is not achievable without good nutrition. Whilst being a biological requirement, there are other benefits associated with eating and drinking. In some cultures, much emphasis is placed on the social aspects of eating and drinking such as the preparation, cooking and eating of food since such tasks can be utilised as quality time for when families get together. Such meetings could also be related to family celebrations, live events, religious rites or national holidays. Additionally, eating and drinking has a psychological aspect as a form of comfort and a feeling of satisfaction. Kozier et al. (2008) suggest that other factors need to be considered in relation to eating and drinking, which include gender, personal preference and beliefs about food, lifestyle and religious beliefs. However, it is important to remember that individuals' beliefs can vary considerably from orthodox to liberal. For example, it is important not to make any assumptions in relation to a person's stated religion as there are considerable differences and practices within the same religion.

Activity 5.2

Consider the following religions and identify what might need to be considered in relation to eating and drinking needs.

Religion	Food considerations	Religious festivals
Christian (including Catholic and Protestant)		
Judaism		
Sikhism		
Hinduism		
Islam		
Seventh Day Adventist		
Jehovah's Witness		
Buddhism		
Agnostic		

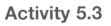

Activity 5.3

Please consider the following foodstuffs and identify if they can be consumed by the given groups (please put a tick in the box if you think it applies).

Food type	Carnivore	Omnivore	Vegetarian	Vegan
Vegetables				
Poultry				
Egg/egg products				
Gelatine				
Fish (with scales)				
Shellfish				
Meat				
Dairy				

Isaac and Isaac (2004) imply that, today, people are considering the importance of how the food they eat keeps them healthy as opposed to keeping them alive. Dunne (2007) suggests that the aim of eating healthily is to achieve the optimum value in terms of calorific energy which can be obtained from the food eaten. Other important aspects to consider also include vitamins, minerals, fats, carbohydrates and protein for the growth and repair of the body. Dunne (2007) points out that a healthy diet does not automatically make us immune to serious diseases but such measures can reduce the threat of developing such diseases. With reference to healthy eating and its calorific content, in more recent times concerns have been raised in the media relating to certain issues associated with eating and drinking. One such concern is the American phenomenon termed 'size zero' (equivalent to size 4 in the UK) which has led to an increase in young people developing eating disorders (Porter, 2007). In contrast, obesity is well publicised in the media with over-nutrition being equally as detrimental as under-nutrition. Reports suggest that 24% of adults and 29.7% of children are obese which could lead to other related conditions such as diabetes mellitus and cardiac disease in later life (DH, 2008). Additionally, many studies have been carried out in relation to malnutrition which, according to Dunne (2007), is a condition used to describe the results as a consequence of poor dietary intake and subsequent lack of nutrients (McWhirter and Pennington, 1994; Lennard-Jones, 1999; Age Concern, 2006). It is essential that nursing interventions provide unfaltering opportunities to meet the nutritional needs of patients. However, certain diseases, disorders or situations may not allow patients to eat or drink in the conventional way.

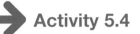 Activity 5.4

Can you identify some diseases or disorders which could prevent people from eating and drinking in the conventional way? Use the space below for your answers.

Activity 5.4 (*Continued*)

Anatomy and physiology associated with eating and drinking

To fully understand the importance of eating and drinking in everyday life, knowledge of the associated anatomy and physiology is essential. Central to the idea of eating and drinking is the digestive system as this system is fundamental to the digestion and conversion of the food and drinks which we consume into energy and hydration for the body's functioning. Energy can be defined as the ability to carry out work (Heath, 1995). Digestion involves the chewing and churning of the food and the breaking down of the food into its simplest form. The rate at which the food is broken down is called metabolism and it relates to all biochemical and physiological processes by which the body grows and maintains itself (Kozier *et al.*, 2008). According to Heath (1995), metabolism consists of two reactions:

- *Anabolic reactions*. The building of body tissue.
- *Catabolic reactions*. The breaking down of substances within the stomach to assist with absorption.

> ## Activity 5.5
>
> **Can you name the following anatomical features and their functions associated with eating and drinking?**
>
>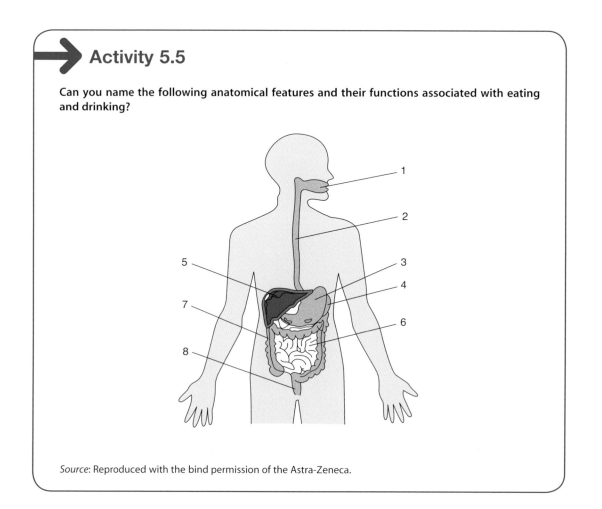
>
> *Source*: Reproduced with the bind permission of the Astra-Zeneca.

When food is swallowed, it is moved along the digestive tract by means of peristalsis. Once it reaches the stomach, it is broken down with the aid of certain enzymes, the main one being pepsin. The broken down food in the stomach is known as chyme and this flows into the duodenum where it mixes with other liquids such as bile, intestinal juices and pancreatic emissions. As the mixture moves along the small intestine, it is further broken down and this is where the absorption of the essential nutrients takes place. These are then transported via the circulatory system throughout the body and usually via the liver. At this time, motility is important as motility relates to the speed in which the mixture moves along the small intestine. If it moves too fast (e.g. if the patient has diarrhoea) or there is malabsorption (e.g. due to ulceration of the small intestine), this could lead to non-absorption of the essential nutrients. Within the large intestine, the only nutrient absorbed is water – this makes the mixture (now known as faeces) more bulky, which then passes along the large intestine to the rectum and through the anus for defaecation or elimination. Chapter 6 discusses elimination in more detail.

→ Activity 5.6

In relation to the anatomical features below, what problems or issues could hinder eating and drinking?

Anatomical feature	Problems or issues
Mouth	
Pharynx	
Epiglottis	
Oesophagus	
Stomach	
Small intestine	
Large intestine	
Rectum	
Anus	

Whilst the gastrointestinal tract is considered to be the standard mechanism for the ingestion and digestion of food and fluids, at times the upper gastrointestinal tract cannot be used. This could be due to neurological issues such as a cerebrovascular accident (CVA or stroke), motor neurone disease or Parkinson's disease. In these situations, dysphagia (impaired ability to swallow food or fluids effectively from the upper gastrointestinal tract into the stomach) may occur. This could lead to further problems such as aspiration (inhaling food and fluid into the lungs) and subsequently cause recurrent chest infections, pneumonia or even death. Such a risk needs to be assessed and determined by a speech and language therapist or a nurse specialist/nurse consultant who are competent in carrying out these assessments. Consequently, advice will be given as to how this situation should be managed.

Activity 5.7

What alternative methods could be used instead of the gastrointestinal tract to ensure that the patient is adequately hydrated and nourished? Use the space below.

The body needs a balanced and adequate nutritional intake in the form of vitamins and minerals to ensure the body's safety as well as relying on a store of nutrients in times of crisis to protect it and in times of sickness to keep it safe from further disease. Grodner *et al.* (2000) define nutrition as the study of essential nutrients and the process by which nutrients are used by the body. Grodner *et al.* (2000) also state that nutrients are substances in foods that are required by the body for energy, growth, maintenance and repair. Metabolism is also essential for the breaking down and storage of nutrients whilst the person is well and also at times of illness (Brogden, 2004). There are two main groups of nutrients which must be considered in relation to eating and drinking and these are macro-nutrients (carbohydrates, proteins and lipids) and micro-nutrients (vitamins and minerals) (Green and Jackson, 2006; Kozier *et al.*, 2008).

Macronutrients

Carbohydrates

Carbohydrates are a primary source of energy for the body and they can be divided into simple carbohydrates (sugars) and complex carbohydrates (starch). Simple carbohydrates are produced naturally in plants and animals and they can be broken down as follows:

- *Monosaccharide*. Known as simple sugars and include glucose and fructose. These are usually found in fruits but they can be found in other foods as well.
- *Disaccharide*. Usually a processed or concentrated form of simple sugar and it includes sucrose (table sugar), lactose (which is found in milk and some milk products) and maltose.
- *Polysaccharide*. Known as a complex carbohydrate and is found in starch and non-starch forms. The starch form is found in foods such as potatoes, cereals, bread, rice and pasta. Non-starch form is also called fibre and this is found in cereal grains such as bran and some vegetables. However, the more refined the food, the less non-starch it contains (Green and Jackson, 2006).

Protein

Protein is essential for the welfare of every cell in the body as it is required for growth. It is also essential for tissue viability and wound repair. Protein is found in a variety of foods including eggs, meat and fish. According to Kozier *et al.* (2008), protein is made up of chains of amino acids of which there are 22 different types:

- Fourteen non-essential amino acids which are not derived from food and they can be produced by the body and are vital for neurotransmitters (which send and receive messages in the brain) and for the metabolism of glucose.
- Eight essential amino acids which are derived from food sources and are essential for the growth and repair of the body.

Protein cannot be stored in the body; therefore, eating too much protein could result in obesity since it can be digested into glucose and used as energy or stored as fat. Additionally, it is important to be aware of a person's protein intake as the excretion of protein may damage certain organs such as the kidneys and the liver.

Lipids

A lipid is a comprehensive term for all fats which are solid at room temperature and oils which are liquid at room temperature (Heath, 1995). Such fats are not soluble in water but soluble in other solvents such as ethanol (alcohol). They are composed of carbon, hydrogen and oxygen molecules. One of the major lipids in the human body is glycerol but other molecules known as fatty acids attach themselves to glycerol. These are referred to as triglycerides and they come in three forms: saturated, unsaturated and polyunsaturated. Saturated and polyunsaturated lipids can hold many hydrogen molecules (a process known as hydrogenation). Unsaturated lipids are limited in the amount of hydrogen they can hold. Most animal fats have high levels of saturated fatty lipids; most vegetable lipids have higher unsaturated and polyunsaturated lipid levels. There is just one essential lipid which the body requires and that is linoleic acid as this is essential for growth but cannot be synthesised by the body (Martin, 2003); this is a polyunsaturated lipid which is found in oils from plants such as sunflower, peanut, corn and soybean.

Micronutrients

Vitamins

A vitamin is an organic compound which cannot be produced by the body and is needed in small quantities to catalyse metabolic processes (Kozier *et al.*, 2008). Therefore, dietary intake is vital for this to happen. It must be noted that food preparation needs to be considered to maintain the vitamin content of food; the vitamin content is usually higher in food which is fresh and has had little exposure to heat, air or water (Heath, 1995). Vitamins are usually classed as water soluble (which cannot be stored in the body and must be derived from dietary intake) or fat soluble (which can be stored in the body). It is essential to note that an excess intake in water-soluble vitamins could lead to hypervitaminosis which can easily happen as a result of a busy lifestyle. The importance of these vitamins is explained in Tables 5.1 and 5.2.

Minerals

According to Kozier *et al.* (2008), minerals are inorganic compounds whose molecules cannot be broken down, changed or destroyed by the body in any way. There are common problems associated with the lack of minerals to include iron deficiency anaemia and osteoporosis to name but two. There are two categories of minerals:

- *Macro-minerals*. Those minerals which people require amounts in excess of 100 milligrams per day.
- *Micro-minerals*. Those minerals which people require amounts less than 100 milligrams per day; these can also be referred to as trace elements.

Information pertaining to both macro- and micro-minerals is outlined in Tables 5.3 and 5.4.

Vitamins and minerals are essential in one way or another to ensure the welfare of the person whilst maintaining health and preventing disease. However, this relies heavily on a healthy diet and adequate intake of fluids. Issues such as malnutrition and serious illness need to be revisited once more since people can experience problems with re-feeding syndrome and its associated concerns with the sudden re-introduction of food after long periods of starvation (Green and Jackson, 2006). With periods of starvation, there is a reduced secretion of insulin due to a reduced intake of carbohydrates; consequently, fat and protein stores are used for energy (Hearing, 2004). With the sudden re-introduction of food, or re-feeding syndrome, the body cannot adapt to such rapid changes. Therefore, food and fluid intake cannot be broken down in the appropriate way as outlined earlier in this chapter and it can also cause other problems such as cardiac failure

Table 5.1   Water-soluble vitamins
(*Source:* Adapted from Heath, 1995 and Green and Jackson, 2006.)

Vitamins and their uses	What may happen if the vitamin is lacking	What may happen if the person has too much of the vitamin	Food sources which can provide the vitamin
B1 (thiamine) Formation of red blood cells Also essential for skin formation	Mental confusion and lack of awareness, weak muscle strength, abnormal heart beat and cardiac enlargement	Rapid pulse, inability to rest and sleep, headaches, irritability	Fish, eggs, poultry, bread, pasta, oatmeal, whole grains, wheat germ
B2 (riboflavin) Breaking down of carbohydrate (which is known as oxidation)	Cracks at the corners of the mouth, intolerance of light (photophobia) which can lead to further eye irritation, glossitis (inflammation of the tongue)	Increased blood glucose and uric acid levels	Milk, liver, green vegetables, whole grains
Niacin Used for tissue repair, protein utilisation, fat synthesis	Anorexia, a general feeling of physical weakness in the body, indigestion, dementia-type presentation to include issues such as confusion, dermatitis, diarrhoea	Increased blood glucose and urea levels, liver dysfunction, nausea	Dairy products, meats, tuna, whole grains, cereals

(*continued*)

Table 5.1   (*Continued*)

Vitamins and their uses	What may happen if the vitamin is lacking	What may happen if the person has too much of the vitamin	Food sources which can provide the vitamin
B6 (pyridoxine) Essential for the metabolism of nutrients, synthesis of non-essential amino acids, functioning of the blood and central nervous system	Anaemia (a reduction in red blood cells which reduces the ability to carry oxygen around the body), irritability, impaired functioning and possible breakdown of the skin	Depression, bloating, nerve damage, irritability	Liver, fish, poultry, green beans, nuts, meats, potatoes
Folic acid Essential for the metabolism of some amino acids, essential for deoxyribonucleic acid (DNA)	Abnormally large red blood cells (macrocytic anaemia), can cause foetal deficiencies in pregnancy, for example spina bifida	Insomnia, depression, diarrhoea, can also mask vitamin B12 deficiency	Green leafy vegetables, meat, fish, poultry, whole grains, liver
B12 (cobalamin) Used for the function of cells of bone marrow, gastrointestinal tract and nervous systems, metabolism of nutrients]	Pernicious anaemia (lack of manufacture of red blood cells which can interfere with bone marrow cells), problems with the central nervous system (to include the brain, spinal cord and peripheral nerves)	None	Cheese, milk, eggs, meat, fish, all other foods of animal origin

Vitamins and their uses	What may happen if the vitamin is lacking	What may happen if the person has too much of the vitamin	Food sources which can provide the vitamin
C (ascorbic acid) Essential for the production of collagen, formation of red blood cells, protection of other vitamins	Poor wound healing, bleeding gums, bruising, tooth loss, scurvy	Kidney stones, urinary tract infections	Citrus fruits, potatoes, cabbage, tomatoes, broccoli, strawberries
Pantothenic acid Required for the metabolism of nutrients, synthesis of cholesterol and steroid hormones, especially the activity of adrenal gland	None	Water retention, occasional diarrhoea	Vegetables, whole grain cereals, meat
Biotin Needed for the synthesis of lipids, utilisation of glucose, vitamin B12 and folic acid, metabolism of protein	None	None	Liver and kidneys of animals, dark green vegetables, egg yolk, green beans

(Hearing, 2004). Therefore, patients will need to be treated by those who possess specialist knowledge, skills and expertise in the requirements of nutritional support (National Institute for Health and Clinical Excellence (NICE), 2006). Specific screening, including biochemistry (blood tests to include levels of glucose, phosphate, nitrogen, magnesium, calcium, potassium, micro-nutrients and electrolytes), physically (blood pressure and pulse, weight, height) and nutritionally (with the aid of nutritional assessment tools), must be carried out at this time. It is recommended

Table 5.2   Fat-soluble vitamins
(*Source:* Adapted from Heath, 1995 and Green and Jackson, 2006).

Different names of vitamins and their uses	What may happen if the vitamin is lacking	What may happen if the person has too much of the vitamin	Food sources which can provide the vitamin
A (retinol) Required for tissue growth and maintenance, immune functions, visual accuracy in dim light	Rough scaly skin, night blindness, dry mucous membranes, prone to infections, incomplete bone and tooth development	Nausea, vomiting, abdominal pain, weight loss in adults, growth failure in children, hair loss, joint and bone pains, liver and spleen problems, headaches	Eggs, whole milk products, liver, fish liver oil, green leafy vegetables
D (cholecalciferol) Required for the absorption of calcium for bone and tooth formation	Osteomalacia in adults (softening of the bones), rickets and dental problems in children	Decreased appetite, growth failure, weight loss, increased calcium in bodily parts such as the kidneys	Fortified milk, sunlight, eggs, meats, cereals
E (tocopherol) Protection of vitamins A and D and polyunsaturated lipids	Macrocytic anaemia	Interference with vitamins A and K utilisation, increased blood clotting time, fatigue, headaches, dizziness	Milk, eggs, cereals, green leafy vegetables, vegetable oils
K Blood clotting, prothrombin formation	Non-clotting of blood in newborn infants, prolonged clotting time in adults	Excessive levels of bilirubin in infants, vomiting in adults	Liver, green leafy vegetables

Table 5.3   The macro-minerals
(*Source:* Adapted from Heath, 1995 and Green and Jackson, 2006).

Different names of minerals and their uses	What may happen if the mineral is lacking	What may happen if the person has too much of the mineral	Food sources which can provide the mineral
Calcium Required for the formation of teeth and bones, contraction of muscle fibres, nerve impulse transmission, cardiac function, coagulation of blood, activation of enzymes	Tingling in extremities such as fingers and toes, muscle cramps, convulsions, pathological fractures even in minor falls and bumps, stunted growth in children	Cardiac irregularities, relaxed skeletal muscles	Milk and milk products, fish, small edible bones, leafy vegetables
Magnesium Required for the maintenance of B vitamins, maintenance of electrical activity in nerves, utilisation of calcium and potassium and protein	Confusion, hallucinations, growth failure, neuromuscular problems	Lethargy, diarrhoea	Nuts, green vegetables, whole grains
Phosphorus Required for the formation of bones and teeth, activation of B vitamins, muscle and nerve activity, metabolism of carbohydrates	Defective white blood cell function, delayed clotting, bone pain, pathological fractures, haemolytic anaemia	Calcium loss, erosion of the jaw	Dried peas and beans, pork, beef, milk and milk products

Table 5.4   The micro-minerals
(*Source:* Adapted from Heath, 1995 and Green and Jackson, 2006).

Different names of minerals and their uses	What may happen if the mineral is lacking	What may happen if the person has too much of the mineral	Food sources which can provide the mineral
Copper Required for haemoglobin formation to allow the transportation of oxygen in the blood, activation of some enzymes	Abnormal blood cell development in infants and bone demineralisation	Dizziness, nausea, headaches, vomiting, diarrhoea, Wilson's disease (deposits of copper in the liver which causes jaundice and cirrhosis, or in the brain which can cause symptoms resembling Parkinson's disease), heartburn	Shellfish, raisins, nuts, offal
Fluoride Essential for the formation of teeth and the prevention of tooth decay	Poor dental health	Mottling, pitting and discolouration of tooth enamel	Seafood, toothpaste, mouthwash, fluorinated water
Iodine Essential for thyroid functioning	Depressed thyroid functioning	Toxic goitre	Seafood, food additives, colouring agents
Iron Essential for the formation of haemoglobin and antibodies, synthesis of vitamins	Anaemia, fatigue, decreased immunity, weakness, lethargy	Cramps, abdominal pains, nausea, vomiting, elimination of black stools, liver cirrhosis	Liver, lean meats, whole grains, green leafy vegetables, enriched breads and cereals

Different names of minerals and their uses	What may happen if the mineral is lacking	What may happen if the person has too much of the mineral	Food sources which can provide the mineral
Zinc Essential for connective tissue (skin) formation and consistency, immune responses, formation of enzymes and insulin	Impaired wound healing, decreased sensation of taste and smell, skin lesions	Anaemia, fever, nausea, vomiting, muscle pain, weakness, decreased calcium absorption	Oysters, liver, poultry, meats, vegetables, nuts

that people who have eaten little or nothing for more than 5 days should have nutrition support introduced at no more than 50% of their requirements for the first 2 days of the re-introduction of food (NICE, 2006). It is also recommended that metabolic and gastrointestinal tolerance of feeding should be observed and reported and documented accordingly.

> ### ➡ Activity 5.8
>
> **Revision time! Try the following questions and put your answers in the space provided.**
>
> | Question | Answer |
> |---|---|
> | What is nutrition? | |
> | Why is nutrition important? | |
> | What is the equivalent UK size for the American 'size zero'? | |
> | According to the Department of Health (2008), what percentage of adults in the UK is obese? | |
> | According to the Department of Health (2008), what percentage of children in the UK is obese? | |
> | What are the two reactions associated with metabolism? | |
>
> *(continued)*

Activity 5.8 (Continued)

Question	Answer
Name the two classifications for vitamins.	
What are the other names for the following vitamins: vitamin B1 vitamin B12 vitamin A vitamin E	
What are the classifications for minerals?	
Name four food sources which are deemed to be rich in iron.	
What may happen if the patient is lacking zinc in his or her diet?	
Why is copper important in the patient's diet?	

Importance of fluid intake

According to Kozier *et al.* (2008), the maintenance of fluid balance within the body is vital for the sustenance of life and they estimate that the total body weight of people consists of between 50% and 70% water. This amounts to approximately 9 L of fluid passing through the adult gastrointestinal tract each day but approximately 7.5 L is reabsorbed. Kozier *et al.* (2008) also suggest that a person would not survive for more than 3 days without water; therefore, the maintenance of fluid levels within the body is essential. Consequently, it is paramount that fluid output and input levels are balanced for the body to function appropriately. The primary method of fluid intake is by drinking but other methods such as intravenous (IV) fluids or artificial feeding are also important. The predominant method of fluid removal from the body is by urinating. However, fluid levels within the body can also decrease through insensible loss such as sweating and breathing (excretion of water vapour – think about exhaling on a cold, frosty morning!). Illness and infection can threaten such a balance as can some medications called diuretics which are used in the treatment of cardiac problems and hypertension. Severe burns can lead to excessive fluid loss and this would need to be rectified accordingly. Conversely, having excess bodily fluid can also be detrimental to the person's welfare as it can lead to problems such as breathlessness, oedema of the extremities (hands and feet) and renal problems. Such problems may require a fluid intake restriction and careful measuring of fluid output.

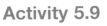

Activity 5.9

Calculate the fluid output and input for the following patients and determine whether the patients have a positive or negative balance of fluid in their system.

Patient name	Input over 24 h	Output over 24 h	Positive/negative balance? Any other issues?
Mr Holweg No fluid restriction	Coffee : 670 mL Tea : 540 mL IV fluids : 2000 mL	Urine : 2400 mL	
Mrs Patel No fluid restriction	Orange juice : 300 mL Tea : 500 mL Water : 250 mL Cola : 250 mL	Urine : 1400 mL	
Mrs Torres 1500 mL fluid restriction	Coffee : 450 mL Ovaltine : 250 mL Water : 750 mL IV fluids : 500 mL	Not measured	
Mr White 1000 mL fluid restriction	Water : 70 mL Tea : 250 mL IV fluids : 500 mL	Urine : 500 mL	

Assessment of eating and drinking needs

Whilst an understanding of the anatomy and physiology and the importance of eating and drinking are essential for care delivery, this information alone is not exclusive to the delivery of optimum care according to the needs of any patient you care for. Nutritional assessment is no different as this is needed to determine the patient's nutritional status which should inform care delivery (Grodner et al., 2000). In addition to this, Grodner et al. (2000) suggest that the **ABCD** approach is effective when caring for the nutritional needs of patients:

- *Anthropometrics.* Body measurements which include height and weight.
- *Biochemical tests.* Routine and specific blood tests and other tests such as urinalysis.
- *Clinical observations.* Observing skin, hair nails, oral cavity, swallowing ability, as well as temperature, pulse, respiratory rate, blood pressure, peripheral blood glucose testing (a drop of blood obtained from the side of the finger) and oxygen saturation levels by means of a probe attached to the finger or toe.
- *Diet evaluation.* Begin with a 24-h food recall and ask the patient to tell you about the beverages and foods which he or she has eaten over the past 24 h. This can also lead to commencing food and fluid charts or records to monitor input.

Whilst the information obtained from the different sources above is helpful and sometimes essential, it must be remembered that the assessment of eating and drinking needs does not rest solely on this information. As previously mentioned, a patient's condition (medical or otherwise) may change whilst in your care; alternatively, important information may come to light and, as a result, measures must be taken to adapt the care delivery accordingly. We have briefly looked at some of the possible physiological issues which may affect eating and drinking ability in Activity 5.4. However, please consider the following activity.

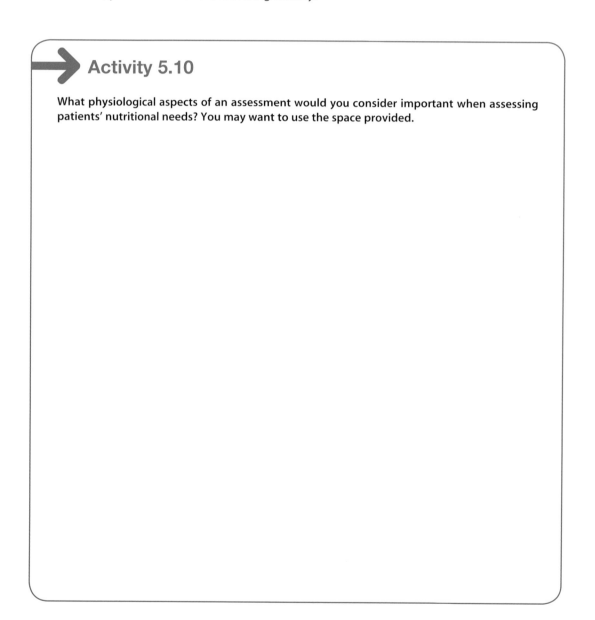

Activity 5.10

What physiological aspects of an assessment would you consider important when assessing patients' nutritional needs? You may want to use the space provided.

According to Dunne (2007), there are other aspects which need to be considered and are equally as important as physiological needs.

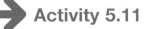 **Activity 5.11**

Under the headings below, what aspects do you think you would need to consider or determine to ensure that you have carried out a comprehensive eating and drinking assessment?

Psychological	Social
Emotional	Other

→ Activity 5.12

Can you think of any sources where you can get information pertaining to the eating and drinking needs of your patients? There is a space provided below for you to write your response if you wish.

Assessment, planning, implementation and evaluation on a cyclical and continuous basis are critical, especially with the patient's changing presentation. Many sources of data will influence the assessment of needs and it is essential that the nurse observes both the verbal and non-verbal information when assessing eating and drinking needs. Any issues which are observed must be reported to the registered nurse and such issues must be documented in the patient's care notes. This information will be used for the evaluation of the patient's care and it could determine the effectiveness, or not, of the nutritional care intervention regimen.

Nutritional screening tools

To further assist healthcare workers in their delivery of optimum care, nutritional screening tools are critical implements used by nurses and other healthcare professionals in identifying those who are most at risk from malnutrition or obesity (Green and McLaren, 1998). Such tools can be used in a variety of settings ranging from inpatient hospital units to community working. Assessment and/or screening tools are many and varied but they must be reliable and valid to measure what is expected of them to identify care needs. Green and McLaren (1998) suggest that these should be easy to use, quick to complete and be easily understood to the patient. One tool, the Body Mass Index (BMI) tool, is often used to determine malnutrition or obesity.

Body mass index

According to NHS Direct (2008a), BMI is a tool which can be used to tell how healthy a person's weight is in relation to his or her height. It is calculated by using the following equation:

- Take your weight (in kilograms (kg)) and divide this by your height (in metres (m)).
- Divide the result of the above by your height (in metres) again.

    For example, a patient weighs 90 kg and he or she is 1.95 m tall. Therefore, 90/1.95 = 46.15 (approx.); 46.15/1.95 = 23.6. The patient's BMI is 23.6. But what does this figure mean? The World Health Organisation (WHO) has specified a determining grade which BMI is measured against:

- BMI < 18.4: patient is underweight for his or her height.
- BMI 18.5–24.9: patient is an ideal weight for his or her height.
- BMI 25–29.9: patient is over the ideal weight for his or her height.
- BMI 30–39.9: patient is obese.
- BMI > 40: patient is very obese.

    It is generally suggested that if a BMI is over 25, then patients should be encouraged to lose weight since serious health issues, such as heart disease and diabetes mellitus, can arise if the patient's weight continues to rise. However, the use of BMI measurement is limiting since the outcome from a BMI measurement tool can only be used in adult care and it does not apply to children (NHS Direct, 2008b). In recent times, the validity of the BMI tool has been questioned. Other issues which need to be considered include the physiological status of the person in question, for example a pregnant woman, a woman who is breastfeeding, a man or woman who is an athlete or weight trainer. Age is also a crucial factor since adulthood is usually determined up to 65 years, as well as other factors associated with long-term conditions. According to Hicks (2005) waist measurement (80 cm for women; 94 cm for men) and waist–hip ratio (waist bigger than hips at a rate of 0.8 for women and 1.0 for men) are better determinants when considering malnutrition or obesity.

→ Activity 5.13

See if you can calculate the following, using the equation above, to determine the patient's BMI score.

Weight: 87 kg; Height: 1.25 m	Weight: 96 kg; Height: 2 m
Weight: 80 kg; Height: 1.34 m	Weight: 65 kg; Height: 1.75 m

    At times, it is not possible to obtain a patient's height, for example through prolonged bed rest or unconsciousness. However, the British Association for Parenteral and Enteral Nutrition (BAPEN) (2008) has suggested alternative methods of obtaining a patient's height. One method is estimating the height of the person from measuring the length of the ulna. The point between the point of the elbow (the olecranon process) and the midpoint of the bony prominence of the wrist (the styloid process) must also be measured. BAPEN has suggested that the left hand is used for measurement. The result of the measurement is then cross-referenced with a nominated graph of results from which the patient's weight can be estimated.

BAPEN (2008) suggest another alternative method of estimating BMI in patients which involves measuring the mid upper arm circumference (MUAC). The patient's arm needs to be bent at the elbow at a 90° angle. The distance between the point of the elbow (the olecranon process) and the bony point of the shoulder (acromion) must be measured and the mid-point determined. The circumference of the mid-point is measured whilst the arm is allowed to hang loose and the result is compared against set criteria as follows:

- MUAC < 23.5 cm; BMI is likely to be <20 kg/m^2.
- MUAC > 32.0 cm; BMI is likely to be >30 kg/m^2 (BAPEN, 2008).

Further information regarding these measurements and other important information pertaining to nutritional needs is available in Figure 5.1. Alternatively, further information

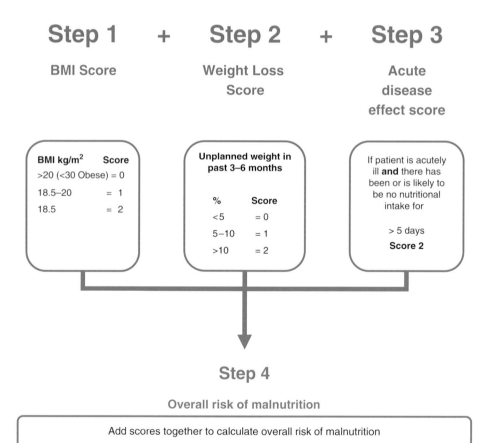

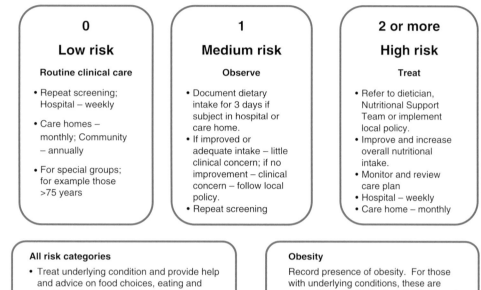

Step 5

Management guidelines

0	1	2 or more
Low risk	**Medium risk**	**High risk**
Routine clinical care	Observe	Treat
• Repeat screening; Hospital – weekly • Care homes – monthly; Community – annually • For special groups; for example those >75 years	• Document dietary intake for 3 days if subject in hospital or care home. • If improved or adequate intake – little clinical concern; if no improvement – clinical concern – follow local policy. • Repeat screening	• Refer to dietician, Nutritional Support Team or implement local policy. • Improve and increase overall nutritional intake. • Monitor and review care plan • Hospital – weekly • Care home – monthly

All risk categories	Obesity
• Treat underlying condition and provide help and advice on food choices, eating and drinking when necessary. • Record malnutrition risk category.	Record presence of obesity. For those with underlying conditions, these are generally controlled before the treatment of obesity.

Figure 5.1   The malnutrition universal screening tool (MUST)
(*Source*: The 'Malnutrition Universal Screening Tool' (MUST) is reproduced here with the kind permission of BAPEN (British Association for Parenteral and Enteral Nutrition)

pertaining to the importance of nutritional needs and measurement guides is available on the BAPEN website: www.bapen.org.uk.

When the required information is obtained, it is essential that those caring for patients with nutritional needs act upon the information received for the welfare of the patient. The Malnutrition Universal Screening Tool (MUST) (Figure 5.1) was developed by the Malnutrition Advisory Group (MAG) of BAPEN and first produced in November 2003. The MUST assessment tool takes into account the results of three components – recent changes in weight, BMI measurement and a measure of acute diseases. The results are then applied to specify nutritional risk and they can be linked to a nutritional care plan. The MUST has been validated for use in the hospital, community and care settings, the evidence base being contained in The 'MUST' report. An explanatory booklet on MUST is also available for use in training and implementation. Copies of both the report and booklet are available from the BAPEN Office at www.bapen.org.uk.

Activity 5.14

What are the roles of the following members of the multidisciplinary healthcare team members considering the nutritional needs of patients?

Team member	Roles
Registered nurse	
Doctor	
Healthcare assistant	
Dietician	
Speech and language therapist	
Nutrition coordinator	

Practicalities of assisting patients with their eating and drinking needs

When considering the importance of eating and drinking, it is essential that healthcare staff take a proactive approach to the nutritional needs of their patients. The Department of Health (2001) in the *Essence of Care* document has highlighted nutrition as one of the essential benchmarks (or quality care initiatives) which needs to be met for all patients admitted to hospitals in the UK. According to Alexander *et al.* (2006), ensuring a supply of nutritious food, at the right temperature and in an attractive and hygienic manner, is the responsibility of the nursing and catering services. Additionally, mealtimes should not be seen as an added burden to the already-laden nurse's workload, but they should be incorporated as a social and therapeutic event. However, such an activity can be fraught with specific or potential dilemmas but, with careful consideration, these should not be insurmountable. One of the principal issues relates to the non-recognition of the identified issues following assessment and the non-conformance to the agreed plan of individualised care (Hayward, 2003). Other concerns relate the non-recognition of the issues which are highlighted in the Case study 5.5 found on the website.

Activity 5.15

What issues need to be considered when exploring at the practicalities of mealtimes within a hospital setting? Record your answers in the space provided.

Activity 5.15 (*Continued*)

When assessing the needs of individual patients, it is worth remembering that the majority of patients will be able to meet their known eating and drinking needs without any assistance from staff when a meal is placed in front of them. However, there are times when a more comprehensive approach is required when meeting the individual's nutritional needs. Below are some pointers which you may need to consider whilst ensuring that your patients will receive optimum care relating to their eating and drinking requirements:

- Be aware of your patient's nutritional needs pertaining to dietary requirements. This will further assist you and your patient in menu choice. If you are unsure, please ask a registered nurse and/or consult the case notes documentation.
- Be aware of any specific medical or surgical reasons as to why your patient is not allowed food or fluids. It may be that your patient is nil by mouth for blood testing, invasive procedures or surgery.
- Always be aware of what your patient can and cannot do for himself or herself. If a patient is able to eat and drink unassisted, ensure that these skills are maintained and that the patient is not deskilled (in anticipation of discharge).
- Prior to mealtimes, always offer your patient the opportunity of hand washing as this may have been overlooked by a previous member of staff. This is particularly important if your patient is on bed rest or immobile and having to rely on the use of urinals or a commode for elimination purposes.
- Additionally, in the interest of health and safety, always ensure that the table space where your patient is going to eat is wiped clean before each meal. In hospitals, everything is placed on bedside tables, ranging from urinals to sputum pots.
- Always offer your patient oral care prior to each meal and insert the patient's dentures, if applicable. If necessary, look inside the mouth to ensure that the oral mucosa is intact; also examine the tongue as this could become 'coated' with the effects of dehydration, oxygen therapy or medications such as antibiotics and steroids. This is when a pen torch is most valuable. Report any findings to the registered nurse and record such findings in the patient's care notes.
- Before serving food to your patients, be aware of your local policy in relation to infection control and health and safety. Ensure that you wear the suggested protective clothing in line with local policy.
- Also consider the above and follow local policy when tending to patients who are being cared for in isolation when delivering food trays, removing food trays, or if you need to stay in the isolation room to assist the patients with their eating and drinking needs.
- The best position for any patient to eat and drink is in the sitting position, preferably in a supportive chair next to a table. For those patients who are on bed rest, ensure that they are positioned safely to enable safe self-feeding or positioned to allow safe feeding by a member of staff.
- Always be aware of what your patient can do for himself or herself. It may be that the patient is able to feed himself or herself but small sachets of butter or marmalade or small cereal packets need to be opened and dispensed or applied accordingly to allow self-feeding to happen.
- Ensure that the patient has the necessary utensils and implements to feed himself or herself taking into account physical disabilities such as arthritis. Consider the use of condiments in line with food restrictions for health reasons such as a low sodium diet
- Observe cultural needs – some patients do not implement but use their fingers instead.

- Observe religious issues, especially when food for patients needs to be unpacked or opened. Clarify with your patient that such an action is acceptable. If it is not acceptable for a nurse to unpack or open the food, family members could be involved in the patient's care to carry out such a task and assist with the feeding of the patient at mealtimes, if applicable.
- Observe other forms of therapy such as oxygen therapy. In some cases, patients are on continuous oxygen therapy via a face mask. Always be aware of this, as the lack of oxygen therapy could be detrimental for any patient's welfare. Liaise with the registered nurse to determine if an alternative method of oxygen delivery could be considered.
- For those patients requiring assistance, always ask as to the patients' preference in taking their food. Does the patient like to take occasional drinks of fluid between intakes of food? Observe fluid restrictions, if any.
- Consider the effects of nutritional supplements on patients as these may suppress the appetite. Conversely, some medications such as steroids, vitamin or iron supplements can enhance the appetite.
- Once finished, offer oral hygiene as well as hand washing. Remove and clean dentures if applicable. Make your patient comfortable.
- Finally, document everything the patient has consumed, especially if the patient has been commenced on food or fluid balance charts. Remember, your documentation is invaluable, as it will be perused by other members of the multidisciplinary team and advising them on their next course of action. Overall, you will be exercising your duties accordingly for the welfare of your patients and you will be perceived as an invaluable member of the multidisciplinary team.

➡ Activity 5.16

Reflect on your placement experience when you cared for patients with nutritional needs. Write in sentences what happened, how you felt and what would you do differently (if anything) next time when you care for someone with who required any assistance.

What happened?

How did it make you feel?

What would you do differently (if anything) next time?

Case studies: Consider the case studies below and discuss some of the issues with your mentor or supervisor at work. You can also find some suggested answers on the website.

The case studies below highlight some significant issues related to eating and drinking and the potential risks associated with assumptions when delivering care. According to Green and Jackson (2006), eating and drinking are fundamental issues for the very sustenance of life; therefore, it should be a natural instinct to ensure that those in our care are adequately hydrated and nourished.

Case study 5.1

As a student mental health nurse, I was asked to assist Ann with her dietary intake. Ann had been admitted with depression and her dietary intake was minimal. Ann's fluid intake was satisfactory but her choices of fluids were water, orange juice and black tea or black coffee. It was a usual lunchtime in the clinical area, with typical food being served and assistance with feeding being carried out. However Ann became very agitated when I was trying to assist her with feeding. Ann began to move her head from side to side whilst repeating the word 'No' over and over again. I asked Ann as to why she was reluctant to eat, but she did not answer. On perusing the admission notes and assessments, all I could uncover was an entry saying 'Eats well'. The next time Ann's husband visited, I asked him if there was any significance to Ann's behaviour. He replied, 'Ann is a vegetarian through personal choice and she has been a vegetarian for 35 years. She does not eat meat, fish or any dairy products.' What issues relating to Ann's care needs are pertinent to this scenario?

Case study 5.2

Whilst working in the clinical area, I always carried a pen torch. I also insisted that all staff had access to a pen torch. In relation to eating and drinking, why is it important for all nursing staff to carry (or have access to) a pen torch?

Case study 5.3

If the patients are nil by mouth for surgery or any other investigative procedure, they are not allowed to have any oral intake of fluids or food prior to the procedure. True or False?

Case study 5.4

Whilst working as a senior staff nurse, a patient was admitted with a chest infection which required intravenous antibiotics and oxygen therapy. I observed a member of staff place a breakfast tray onto a patient's bedside table and walk away. What issues relating to this scenario are not conducive to the eating and drinking needs of the patient?

Case study 5.5

Please read the scenario given to see if you can identify any problems or issues.
Whilst working as a charge nurse in a stroke rehabilitation setting, Mary was admitted to the clinical area with pronounced right-sided weakness, which was Mary's dominant side, following a stroke. One morning, I observed a member of staff asking Mary as to what she would like for breakfast. Mary replied that she would like some toast with butter and marmalade. The butter and marmalade were issued in plastic sachets. The staff member duly obliged; she brought the tray to Mary's bedside with the toast on a plate and two unopened sachets of butter and marmalade. The staff member duly left the tray on Mary's bedside table and walked away.
What are the actual and potential problems associated with this case study?

Chapter summary

Adequate nutrition, primarily in the form of eating and drinking, is essential for the very sustenance of life. A person needs to have a balanced intake of vitamins and minerals to ensure that the body can remain well and to successfully defend the body in times of illness and infection. Whilst it is recognised that problems do exist regarding issues pertaining to obesity, conversely there is increasing pressure from other sources such as the media to conform to what society suggests as to what people should look like. In addition to this, other studies have explored the nutritional needs of those who have been admitted to hospitals and care facilities and such studies and government policies and initiatives suggest that the nutritional needs of all patients is of paramount importance.

It is essential that a multidisciplinary approach to the nutritional needs of the patients in our care is adopted and comprehensively implemented. Primarily, nursing staff are pivotal in the implementation of such needs in line with national and local policy. Adherence to locally agreed initiatives is essential as is the fundamental delivery of research-based nutritional care. Additionally, nurses' awareness of patient's needs, via appropriate assessment and subsequent care implementation, will justly reinforce nurses' unique position within the multidisciplinary team whilst being accountable and responsible for their actions. As a result, all nurses must embrace this and any future developments in the field of nutritional assessment strategies and to reclaim nutrition as a key element of effective nursing care.

Answers to Activities

→ Activity 5.1 Key terms

Before discussing the issues associated with eating and drinking, it is essential to understand key terms. Use a dictionary and other literature to find a definition for each of the following key terms. Alternatively, you can discuss the following terms with other healthcare professionals such as registered nurses, doctors and dieticians.

Term	Definition
Nutrition	The study of food in relation to the physiological processes that depend on its absorption by the body.
Malnourishment	The condition caused by an improper balance between what an individual eats and what is required to maintain health.
Kilocalorie	Equivalent to 1000 calories; this unit is used to indicate the energy value of foods. However, other terminology used for kilocalories is kilojoules.
Obesity	The condition in which excess fat has accumulated in the body.
Diet	The foods and drinks that a person regularly consumes. It can also relate to a specific allowance of foods and drinks, or a selection of foods and drinks.
Mastication	The process of chewing food to allow the safe swallowing of food and to allow the further breaking down of food in the alimentary canal.
Digestion	The process in which ingested food is broken down in the alimentary canal into a form which can be absorbed and assimilated by the tissues of the body.
Absorption	The uptake of digested food from the intestine into the blood and lymphatic systems.
Metabolism	The sum of all the chemical and physical changes that take place within the body and enable its continued growth and functioning.
Dehydration	Loss or deficiency of water in the body tissues.
Intestine	The part of the alimentary canal that extends from the stomach to the anus. Also known as the bowel or gut and has two parts: small intestine and large intestine.
Electrolyte	A solution which produces ions which makes the solution more chemically active. Examples include sodium, potassium, chlorine and bicarbonate, to name but a few. In nursing and medical terms, the concentration of separate ions in the circulating blood are is essential for the body's welfare.

Activity 5.1 (*Continued*)

Peristalsis	A wavelike movement that progresses along some of the hollow muscular tubes of the body, such as the intestines. It occurs involuntarily, induced by distension of the walls of the tube. Alternate contraction and relaxation of the circular and longitudinal muscles tends to push the contents of the tube forward.
Chyme	The semiliquid acid mass that is the form in which food passes from the stomach to the small intestine. It is produced by the action of gastric juice and the churning of the stomach.
Stomach	A distensible sac-like organ that forms part of the alimentary canal between the oesophagus and the duodenum.
Nitrogen	Usually a gaseous element and the major constituent of air. It is also an essential constituent of proteins and nucleic acids and is obtained by humans in the form of protein-containing foods. Nitrogenous waste is excreted as urea.
Magnesium	A metallic element which is essential for the proper functioning of muscle and nervous tissue.
Calcium	A metallic element that is an important constituent of bones, teeth and blood. It is also essential for many metabolic processes, including nerve function, muscle contraction and blood clotting.
Potassium	A mineral element and an important constituent of the human body. It is the main base ion of intracellular fluid. High concentrations can lead to kidney failure and irregular heart rate which could result in cardiac arrest.
Assessment	The first stage of the nursing process, in which data about the patient's health status are collected and from which a nursing care plan may be devised.
Carnivorous	Any other animal or plant that feeds on animals. Can be used to describe humans whose diet consists mainly of meat.
Omnivorous	Eating food of both animal and vegetable origin, or any type of food indiscriminately.
Vegetarian	A person who eats food which consists of vegetables and fruit and, probably, some products such as cheese, eggs and milk (usually described as lacto-vegetarians). Some vegetarians may eat fish — this would need to be discussed with individuals.
Vegan	A person who refrains from using any animal products whatsoever for food, clothing or any other purpose.
Halal	Meat from animals which have been killed in accordance with Muslim law.

(*continued*)

Activity 5.1 (*Continued*)

Term	Definition
Kosher	All food which has been prepared and is fit for use in accordance with the laws of Judaism.
Orthodox	Conforming with established or accepted standards, as in religion, behaviour or attitudes.
Diffusion	The mixing of one liquid or gas with another by the random movement of their particles.
Osmosis	The passage of a solvent from one from a less concentrated to a more concentrated solution through a semipermeable membrane. In living organisms, the process of osmosis plays an important role in controlling the distribution of water.
Intracellular	Situated or occurring inside a cell.
Extracellular	Situated or occurring outside a cell.
Oedema	The excessive accumulation of fluid in the body tissues causing parts of the body to swell. Also known as dropsy. Diuretics are usually administered to remove excess fluid.
Diuretic	A drug that increases the volume of urine produced and helps to excrete salts and water from the kidney. There are different types of diuretics: loop diuretics prevent the reabsorption of sodium and potassium in the Loop of Henle; potassium-sparing diuretics prevent excessive loss of potassium; thiazide diuretics prevent the reabsorption of sodium and potassium in the distal kidney tubules.
Homeostasis	The physiological processes by which the internal systems of the body are maintained at equilibrium, despite variations in the external conditions.

Activity 5.2

Consider the following religions and identify what might need to be considered in relation to eating and drinking needs.

Religions and identification of what needs to be considered in relation to eating and drinking (Adapted from Grodner *et al.*, 2000)

Religion	Food and drink considerations	Religious festivals
Christianity (including	Can be both vegetarian and non-vegetarian.	Christmas Easter

Activity 5.2 (Continued)

Catholic and Protestant)	Some Orthodox Christians will not eat meat on a Friday and will fast during Lent. Fish is sometimes the preferred food on a Friday.	Lent (Starts on Ash Wednesday and finishes on Easter Sunday for a period of 40 days). Two main days within include Ash Wednesday and Good Friday. Christians usually eat three small meals on each of the aforementioned which must not include meat of any kind, but foods such as fish and eggs are allowed.
Judaism	Can be vegetarian and non-vegetarian. Orthodox Jews adhere strictly to their dietary laws and will only eat meat which is Kosher. This is meat that is prepared in a special way in accordance to religious laws. Food must be cooked and served separately. Pork and shellfish may not be eaten. Meat and dairy foods are not eaten together. Liberal Jews will have an individual preference and eat a variety of foods. Kosher meals are available in some clinical areas.	Passover (an 8-day holiday where unleavened bread is eaten). Yom Kippur (Day of Atonement, when some Jews fast). The Sabbath is from sunset on Friday to sunset on Saturday.
Sikhism	Can be vegetarian and non-vegetarian. Food must be cooked and served separately.	Diwali or Deepawali
Hinduism	Lacto-vegetarian and vegan vegetarian. Animal foods of beef, pork, lamb and poultry are not eaten. Food must be cooked and served separately.	Diwali or Deepawali
Islam	Can be vegetarian or non-vegetarian. Islam is the religion of the Muslims and they have strict dietary rules. Orthodox Muslims eat no pork products; however, all other meat is allowed if it is 'Halal'. Halal meat is prepared in a specific way according to Muslim law. Food must be cooked and served separately.	May include fasting during Ramadan; fasting is usually from sunrise to sunset.

(continued)

Activity 5.2 (*Continued*)

Religion	Food and drink considerations	Religious festivals
Seventh Day Adventist	Some followers can be vegetarian — both lacto and vegan. Religion prohibits pork and pork-related products, shellfish, alcohol, coffee and tea.	Seventh Day Adventists celebrate the same festivals as the Christian religion (Christmas and Easter). Seventh Day Adventists believe that the Sabbath day was on Saturday; hence they keep Saturday as the day of worship. Work and secular activities are avoided and observance is mandatory. Sabbath begins on Friday evening and continues through to Saturday evening.
Jehovah's Witness	Can be vegetarian or non-vegetarian.	Jehovah's Witnesses follow the Hebrew calendar and they celebrate the death of Jesus in late March/April. Witnesses do not celebrate other Christian festivals or birthdays and may not wish to attend Christmas or birthday festivities. Witnesses respect the right of others to celebrate birthdays but choose not to share in the celebrations. It is believed that although considered a harmless secular custom today, birthday celebrations are actually rooted in paganism. Likewise, they do not celebrate the birthday of Christ.
Buddhism	Can be vegetarian or non-vegetarian.	Saindran Memorial Day — January Parinirvana — February Magha Puja Day — February/March Honen Memorial Day — March Buddha Day (Vesak or Visakah Puja) — May The Ploughing Festival — May Buddhist New Year Varies according to tradition

Activity 5.2 (*Continued*)

		Asalha Puja Day (Dhamma Day) — July Ulambana (Ancestor Day) — July Abhidhamma Day – October Kathina Day — October The Elephant Festival — November Loy Krathorg — December Bodhi Day — December Uposatha — weekly on the lunar quarter day Avalokitesvara's Birthday.
Agnostic	Can be both vegetarian and non-vegetarian. No specific issues.	No recognition of religious festivals.

Activity 5.3

Please consider the following foodstuffs and identify if they can be consumed by the given groups (please put a tick in the box if you think it applies).

Food Type	Carnivore	Omnivore	Vegetarian	Vegan
Vegetables		✓	✓	✓
Poultry	✓	✓		
Egg / Egg products	✓	✓		
Gelatine	✓	✓		
Fish (with scales)	✓	✓		
Shellfish	✓	✓		
Meat	✓	✓		
Dairy	✓	✓	✓	

> ## Activity 5.4

Can you identify some diseases or disorders which could prevent people from eating and drinking in the conventional way? Use the space below for your answers.

Disorders/diseases	Implications for eating and drinking
Disorders of the central nervous system	
Cerebrovascular accident (CVA) or stroke Parkinson's disease, including drooling motor neurone disease Unconsciousness Confusion related to dementias such as Alzheimer's disease	Dysphagia – difficulty with swallowing. Inability to maintain a safe airway. The patient may not be able to feed himself/or herself independently due to the severity of the disease and may require assistance. Inability to concentrate on the task of eating and drinking. Also, the patient may be disorientated in time and place and may not be aware that it is time for meals.
Disorders of the gastrointestinal (GI) tract	
Tumours (cancer) or strictures (obstructions) in any part of the GI tract Perforated bowel Ulceration of the stomach Crohn's disease Ulcerative colitis Gastro-oesophageal reflux disorder (GORD) — regurgitation of food either through the oesophagus or nasal passages Heartburn A feeling of having to clear the throat constantly	Can lead to decreased ability to swallow food and fluids, especially following some treatments such as radiotherapy as fistulae may occur. Ulceration of the stomach may cause nausea and, in extreme situations, vomiting. Crohn's disease is an extreme GI disease and it can affect any part of the GI tract from the mouth to the anus. Should this happen, the patients would need to be seen by a dietician to ensure adequate intake and absorption of the essential nutrients for the food which they eat.
Disorders of the endocrine system	
Diabetes mellitus	Diabetes mellitus relates to the disorder which results in the non-formation of insulin in the pancreas. Insulin is used to break down sugar within the blood following meals. There are two types of diabetes mellitus: Type 1 (insulin-dependent) diabetes mellitus, and Type 2 (non-insulin dependent) diabetes mellitus (Walsh, 2003). This can lead to hypoglycaemia (low blood sugar) which, if left untreated, can be fatal. Conversely, hyperglycaemia (high blood sugar) can be encountered during periods of infection

Activity 5.4 (*Continued*)

	or illness and, if left untreated, can also be fatal. Blood glucose monitoring is therefore essential. Please be aware of the sugar content of foods, especially hidden sugar in processed foods.
Diabetes insipidus	Diabetes insipidus is characterised by large volumes of urinary (polyuria) and extreme thirst (polydipsia). According to Walsh (2003), urine output can range from 5 to 20 L per day. This can lead to dehydration, muscle cramps, headaches and possible decreased blood plasma (hypovolaemia), which can lead to shock. Strict fluid balance recording is essential, whilst clinical observations, skin integrity and daily weight are also vital in treating this situation.
Addison's disease	This occurs when the adrenal gland does not produce enough cortisol (a steroid essential for metabolic activity and energy production). This can lead to hypoglycaemia, anorexia, nausea, weight loss, abdominal pain, dehydration, increased potassium levels, decreased sodium levels and hypotension (low blood pressure) (Walsh, 2003).
Cushing's disease	This occurs when the adrenal gland produces too much cortisol. This causes hyperglycaemia, weight gain, oedema, decreased potassium, increased sodium, hypertension and abdominal discomfort (Walsh, 2003).
Renal disorders	
Pertains to disorders of the kidneys and would include issues such as those patients who need for dialysis	The kidneys are essential for the removal of waste products of metabolism via urine (Selfe, 2006). However, people who require dialysis may have a strict fluid intake regime since the kidneys are not functioning to their optimum level and cannot remove waste matter as quickly as the body requires the kidneys to do so. If the patient takes in too much fluid and does not excrete this excess fluid, this could cause fluid overload which could lead to difficulties in breathing, cardiac problems and mobility (to name but a few).

(*continued*)

Activity 5.4 (*Continued*)

Disorders/diseases	Implications for eating and drinking
Surgery	
Head and neck surgery Gastrointestinal surgery such as formation of a colostomy or ileostomy following a cancer diagnosis Any extensive or prolonged surgery where the patient requires admission to a critical care area such as intensive care Removal of tonsils and/or adenoids Effects of anaesthesia	Patients may be unconscious or may not be able to maintain a safe environment in relation to their airway or their ability to swallow. It could be painful for the person to swallow, especially with the removal of tonsils. With gastrointestinal surgery, the formation of a colostomy or ileostomy may alter the types and consistency of foods and fluids which the patient can now partake of. Anaesthetics can make the person feel nauseous but anaesthetics can also cause dehydration which could require the rapid replacement of essential fluids.
Other causes	
Major trauma or infections such as burns Malnutrition on admission The need to build up the patient's nutritional status prior to surgical intervention Persistent nausea and vomiting as a result of other medical interventions such as chemotherapy Medications Hospital-acquired infections Recurrent chest infections	If a patient has experienced severe burns, then the patient will have lost vast amounts of essential fluids such as plasma. These need to be replenished as soon as possible. Additionally, if the burns are that extensive, it is highly likely that the patient will be sedated, hence unconscious. At times, it is essential to build some patients up as they have been neglecting themselves prior to admission and essential medical or surgical interventions cannot be carried out accordingly as the person could be at risk. Some therapies such as chemotherapy yields unwanted side effects such as nausea as do all medications. It is essential that patients are made aware of these (Roberts, 2007).

Activity 5.4 (*Continued*)

Electrolyte and acid–base balances	
Hyponatraemia – low serum (blood) sodium level Hypernatraemia – high serum sodium level	With hyponatraemia, medical staff may decide to increase the serum sodium level with sodium chloride intravenous infusion but regular venous blood testing will be essential by the appropriate healthcare personnel. With hypernatraemia, assessment of orientation level is essential since disorientation and restlessness are signs of this. Fluids need to be encouraged as well as strict input/output chart. Diet must not include high sodium content — please be aware of this with processed foods.
Hypokalaemia — low serum potassium level Hyperkalaemia — high serum potassium level	With hypokalaemia, potassium can be replaced intravenously via bags of intravenous fluids only. Please monitor IV site for inflammation. Encourage potassium-rich foods, such as bananas, and also note if the patient is taking diuretics or laxatives. With severe hyperkalaemia, the usual treatment is glucose and insulin and will require careful cardiac monitoring (Kozier *et al.*, 2008). Clinical observations essential and please follow all instructions given as per medical staff.
Hypocalcaemia — low serum calcium level Hypercalcaemia — high serum calcium level	Hypocalcaemia is usually treated with oral calcium supplements. Please observe clinical observations and cardiac monitoring. With hypercalcaemia, fluids must be encouraged, and be aware of patient safety, especially in relation to the possibility of fractures. Fibre must be encouraged to prevent constipation and juices (such as cranberry and prune) should be encouraged to remove excess calcium from the kidneys (Kozier *et al.*, 2008).

Activity 5.5

Can you name the following anatomical features and their functions associated with eating and drinking?

Number	Anatomical feature	Function
1	Mouth	Usual point of entry for food and drink. Used to break down and soften food to facilitate the swallowing of food in a safe fashion.
2	Oesophagus	The passage which takes food to the stomach from the pharynx. This is also known as the gullet.
3	Stomach	The place where food and fluids are broken down further with the aid of acids to assist with the absorption of nutrients. Closely linked to the stomach are the liver, the gallbladder (stores bile which is produced by the liver) and the pancreas.
4	Pancreas	Produces enzymes which are used to further break down food in the small intestine.
5	Liver	Absorbs and processes nutrients and detoxifies any harmful substances.
6	Small intestine	Where food is further broken down and the nutrients are absorbed. These nutrients will be further refined and stored in the liver.
7	Large intestine	Soaks up excess water from the broken down food to allow the formation of faeces.
8	Rectum	Where waste matter can be stored until it can be excreted.

Activity 5.6

In relation to the anatomical features below, what problems or issues could hinder eating and drinking? (Suggested answers adapted from Kozier *et al.*, 2008 and Say, 2005b)

Anatomical feature	Problems or issues
Mouth	Swollen or cracked lips Cracks along the side of the mouth Infection of the oral mucosa due to dehydration or inappropriate oral hygiene, which can lead to mouth ulcers Glossitis (white covering of the tongue) due to inappropriate oral hygiene or the effects of medication Swollen tongue due to anaphylaxis (reaction to an allergen); trauma or surgery Ill-fitting dentures or loose teeth due to other issues such as receding gums Gums which are inflamed or bleeding due to inappropriate oral hygiene or infection Oral surgery for tooth extraction Disorders such as oral cancer The effects of hyperemesis (excessive vomiting over a prolonged period) due to infection, food poisoning or even pregnancy
Pharynx	Throat surgery such as a tonsillectomy (removal of tonsils) Infections — sore throat, coughs, colds, flu Tenderness following intubation (the passing of a tube through the mouth and down the pharynx into the lungs to assist patients with artificial breathing, if needed) or extubation (removal of the aforementioned tube) Nasogastric tubes which are inserted through the nose and pass through the pharynx, oesophagus and into the stomach. These are used for artificial feeding, hydration and the administration of medicines. Nasogastric tubes can be fine bore (thin) or large bore (thick) The effects of hyperemesis (excessive vomiting over a prolonged period)
Epiglottis	Neurological disorders — cerebrovascular accident (CVA or stroke), motor neurone disease, Parkinson's disease, multiple sclerosis. Such disorders can result in the loss of muscle tone and reaction time in the mechanical closure of the epiglottis when swallowing, which protects the lungs from aspiration (inhaling of food and fluids into the lungs), which can lead to infections such as pneumonia or, in severe cases, death
Oesophagus	Physical disorders such as ulcers and cancer Hyperemesis Gastro-oesophageal reflux disorder (GORD) — the over production of gastric acid which results in the acid leaking from the stomach into the oesophagus Nasogastric tubes

(continued)

Activity 5.6 (Continued)

Anatomical feature	Problems or issues
Stomach	Physical disorders such as ulcers, inflammation of the lining of the stomach and cancer Hyperemesis (excessive vomiting) Percutaneous endoscopic gastrostomy (PEG) tube which is introduced through the wall of the stomach to be used for feeding. This is usually used when the epiglottis is not functioning and the traditional swallowing food and fluids has been deemed unsafe Gastrointestinal disturbances such as nausea which is a common side effect of medications such as antibiotics, steroids and antidepressants
Small intestine	Diarrhoea which can lead to abdominal cramps and pain You may need to consider another form of feeding called nasojejunal feeding, where a tube is passed via the nose through the pharynx and stomach and into the jejunum Effects of medications such as laxatives
Large intestine	Diarrhoea Hospital acquired infections such as Clostridium Difficile (excessive diarrhoea) Too much absorption of water from breaking down due to peripheral dehydration, leading to the formation of harder faeces Cancer Effects of medications such as laxatives, which can cause cramps and a bloated feeling Stoma formation due to cancer, trauma from bowel surgery or investigations such as a colonoscopy
Rectum	Too much absorption of water from faeces which makes the faeces harder to eliminate Cancer Haemorrhoids (otherwise known as piles) Discomfort following surgical investigations/procedures
Anus	Cancer Haemorrhoids Constipation Discomfort following surgical investigations/procedures

Activity 5.7

What alternative methods could be used instead of the gastrointestinal tract to ensure that the patient is adequately hydrated and nourished? Use the space below.

Methods of ensuring adequate hydration and nourishment	Rationale
Intravenous infusion (IVI)	Fluids such as sodium chloride, glucose and potassium can be administered via a cannula which is inserted into a vein. IV infusions are particularly effective for ensuring adequate levels of fluids to keep the patient hydrated. If a person is not adequately hydrated, this has implications for the other bodily systems such as the cardiac system. IV administration is not without its difficulties and it needs careful monitoring since confused or aggressive patients may proceed to pull the cannula out of the vein.
Enteral feeding (includes nasogastric (NG) feeding, Percutaneous endoscopic gastrostomy (PEG) feeding and percutaneous endoscopic jejunostomy (PEJ) feeding)	Usually used when patients cannot swallow for whatever reason. An NG tube can be used as a short-term measure; PEG and PEJ feeding are used on a longer term basis (Kozier *et al.*, 2008). All methods are effective in ensuring that patients are adequately hydrated and nourished as NG, PEG and PEJ methods allow fluids (such as water) and liquid food supplements to be administered. Medications can also be administered in this way provided that they are water soluble or in liquid form. However, all methods are not without their problems as the patient runs a high risk of aspiration (vomiting the contents of the stomach and inhaling the vomit into the lungs). This can happen since the stomach has to deal with a high volume of fluids as opposed to the usual mixture of fluids and solids. NG tubes can also

(continued)

Activity 5.7 (*Continued*)

Methods of ensuring adequate hydration and nourishment	Rationale
	be prematurely displaced by patients (Pancorbo-Hidalgo *et al.*, 2001). Patients must be sat upright for all procedures and (especially for the NG route) the position of the tube must be determined by a registered nurse prior to commencing administration of fluids through the NG tube. However, once infusion of the fluids and/or fluids has commenced, should the patient vomit, sneeze harshly or start to cough incessantly, stop the fluid administration immediately. **The position of the tube must be rechecked by a registered nurse or other qualified personnel at this point,** since the tube could have become dislodged with the vomiting, coughing or sneezing (National Patient Safety Agency, 2005).
Subcutaneous infusion (S/C)	A means of administering fluids via a cannula under the skin. However, please note that this method is used a last resort, especially if no veins can be found in the patient (e.g. shutdown of the extremities and veins due to hypovolaemic shock (low circulating blood in the body – blood is diverted for use in the major organs to ensure that these keep working) or hypothermia (low body temperature)).
Parenteral nutrition (PN)	Also known as total parenteral nutrition (or TPN). A method of ensuring essential fluid and liquid food administration in those patients who are extremely ill, due to obstruction, trauma, malnutrition, and malabsorption of nutrients, and so on. Usually administered via a catheter into the superior vena cava in the heart. Extreme caution must be utilised with this method of feeding as infection can occur if strict aseptic technique is not observed during the procedure for attaching the PN to the patient (Kingsbury, 1999).

Activity 5.8

Revision time! Try the following questions and put your answers in the space provided.

Question	Answer
What is nutrition?	The study of food in relation to the physiological processes that depend on its absorption by the body (McFerran & Martin, 2003).
Why is nutrition important?	Nutrition involves a specific course of action by which cells receive and use food material or nutrients to support and maintain metabolism in all parts of the body (Say, 2005a).
What is the equivalent UK size for the American 'size zero'?	UK size 4.
According to the Department of Health (2008), what percentage of adults in the UK is obese?	Reports suggest that 24% of adults are obese (Department of Health, 2008.
According to the Department of Health (2008), what percentage of children in the UK is obese?	Reports suggest that 29.7% of children are obese (Department of Health, 2008).
What are the two reactions associated with metabolism?	Anabolic reactions, the building of body tissue; and catabolic reactions, the breaking down of substances within the stomach to assist with absorption.
Name the two classifications for vitamins.	Fat-soluble vitamins Water-soluble vitamins

What are the other names for the following vitamins:
    vitamin B1
    vitamin B12
    vitamin A
    vitamin E
	vitamin B1 – Thiamine
	vitamin B12 – Cobalamin
	vitamin A – Retinol
	vitamin E – Tocopherol

What are the classifications for minerals?	Macro-minerals Micro-minerals
Name four food sources which are deemed to be rich in iron.	Liver, lean meats, green leafy vegetables, whole grains, enriched bread and cereals
What may happen if the patient is lacking zinc in his or her diet?	The patient may experience delayed wound healing, decreased sense of taste and smell, or skin lesions.
Why is copper important in the patient's diet?	Copper is important for the formation of red blood cells to transport oxygen and for the activation of some enzymes.

Activity 5.9

Calculate the fluid output and input for the following patients and determine whether the patients have a positive or negative balance of fluid in their system.

Patient name	Input over 24 h	Output over 24 h	Positive/negative balance? Any other issues?
Mr Holweg No fluid restriction	Coffee — 670 mL Tea — 540 mL IV fluids — 2000 mL	Urine — 2400 mL	Total input = 3210 mL Total output = 2400 mL Positive balance of 810 mL
Mrs Patel No fluid restriction	Orange Juice — 300 mL Tea — 500 mL Water — 250 mL Cola — 250 mL	Urine — 1400 mL	Total input = 1300 mL Total output = 1400 mL Negative balance of 100 mL
Mrs Torres 1500 mL fluid restriction	Coffee — 450 mL Ovaltine — 250 mL Water — 750 mL IV fluids — 500 mL	Not measured	Total input = 1950 mL Total output = Unknown A positive or negative balance cannot be determined in this situation since the urine output has not been measured. This is not appropriate since it is noted that Mrs Torres is on a 1500 mL fluid restriction; hence the non-measurement of output could have detrimental effects on Mrs Torres's general health.
Mr White 1000 mL fluid restriction	Water — 70 mL Tea — 250 mL IV fluids — 500 mL	Urine — 500 mL	Total input = 820 mL Total output = 500 mL Positive balance of 320 mL Since Mr White is on a 1000 mL fluid restriction, he already has a positive balance of 320 mL of fluid in his body. Ideally, with fluid restriction, the amount excreted should be the same as the amount consumed. Therefore, the following day's fluid balance chart for Mr White must contain this information and the following day's intake must be restricted to 680 mL intake to redress the 1000 mL restriction.

Activity 5.10

What physiological aspects of an assessment would you consider important when assessing patients' nutritional needs? You may want to use the space provided. (Adapted from Kozier et al., 2008 and Bennett, 2003)

General appearance — does the patient look tired or listless?

What is the patient's weight — evidence of obesity or anorexia?

Skin — is there evidence of regular skin elasticity (when the skin is pinched, does it 'bounce' back into shape?) Is the skin dry and flaky? Is there evidence of lesions or any other problems such as pressure sores?

Hair — dull/bright/brittle/wispy?

Eyes — dry/dull/evidence of redness?

Lips — dry/cracked?

Tongue — dry/swollen/coated?

Gums — evidence of bleeding/inflamed/swollen/ill-fitting dentures/loose teeth?

Muscle tone — evidence of muscle wasting/flaccid muscles/wasted muscles?

Any other evidence of problems — weakness due to strokes, Parkinson's disease, multiple sclerosis, motor neurone disease?

Activity 5.11

Under the headings below, what aspects do you think you would need to consider or determine to ensure that you have carried out a comprehensive eating and drinking assessment?

Psychological	Social
Affective disorders which relate to the person's mood and can include depression or mania or both	Amounts of food and drinks which are normally taken by the patient
Olfactory or gustatory delusions (respectively thinking that food or drinks smell or taste as if they are poisoned)	Ability to cook for himself or herself
Paranoid states	What is the patient's appetite like at this time?
Confusion and disorientation in time, place and person	Shopping
Inability to concentrate	Ability to function cooking appliances (electric or otherwise)
Stress	Does the person live alone or with somebody else?
	Financial issues

(continued)

Activity 5.11 (*Continued*)

Anxiety — which can lead to nausea and/or vomiting Anorexia nervosa Bulimia Alcohol withdrawal symptoms Drug abuse Self-esteem and how the person views himself or herself	Responsibilities in relation to dependents/pets/family members Other social circumstances prior to admission How does the patient normally spend his or her day? Current or previous employment Any hobbies or pastimes Does the patient use utensils or implements to eat and drink or does he or she like to use his or her fingers? Fine hand-to-mouth coordination without the reprisals of spilling or dropping foods How does the patient feel about eating and drinking in front of others? Is the person a smoker and, if so, what does he or she smoke (cigarettes, cigars, pipe)?
Emotional Does the patient enjoy mealtimes and look forward to these? Does the patient think that he or she has a problem with eating and drinking? Has anything changed in recent times in relation to eating and drinking which make the patient feel upset? Has there been any alteration to the person's ability to eat and drink socially without fear of making an error which could be classed as foolish? If the patient depends on others to meet his or her eating and drinking needs, what are the person's thoughts and feelings about that? Does the patient feel vulnerable and, if so, how does this vulnerability manifest itself? Does the patient want to continue to live and/or is a refusal to eat a method of self-control in relation to maintaining life? What is the patient's own view of his or her situation at this time?	**Other** Any known food or other allergies Likes and dislikes of food and drink Does the patient like 'wet' or 'dry' food? Level of ability to taste or smell food and drinks General appearance of the person Evidence of dehydration, for example flaky skin Body weight on admission — look for signs of recent weight loss, for example jewellery such as a ring slipping off a finger Body height Oral cavity — evidence of damage to the oral mucosa, ill-fitting dentures, odour from breath, ability to chew food, and so on. Skin lesions Cultural and religious implications Therapeutic dietary requirements, for example low sodium, high fibre, high protein, and so on. Pain Medication Cancers/radiotherapy Level of mobility and body strength 'All hospital food is inedible'

Activity 5.12

Can you think of any sources where you can get information pertaining to the eating and drinking needs of your patients? There is a space provided below for you to write your response if you wish.

Patient	Observing the physical status Use of communication with the patient to find out what the needs are Non-verbal communication in what you can see at the time
Family	This can also include friends and neighbours who know the patient in question Information surrounding eating habits and so on is essential
Healthcare team members	General practitioner Community nurses (including healthcare assistants) Practice nurses Day Care staff Dieticians Occupational therapists Social workers Speech and language therapists Medical staff Ward-based nursing staff (including healthcare assistants) who may know the patient from previous experiences/admissions
Healthcare records	Past and present records may give some relevant data pertinent to the situation at this time
Other records	As above Patient-held community records Discharge letters from previous admissions Day Care/Day Hospital records General practitioner records

Activity 5.13

See if you can calculate the following, using the equation above, to determine the patient's BMI score.

Weight: 87 kg; Height: 1.25 m 87/1.25 = 69.6 69.6/1.25 = 55.68	**Weight: 96 kg; Height: 2 m** 96/2 = 48 48/2 = 24
Weight: 80 kg; Height: 1.34 m 80/1.34 = 59.7 59.7/1.34 = 44.55	**Weight: 65 kg; Height: 1.75 m** 65/1.75 = 37.14 37.14/1.75 = 21.22

Activity 5.14

What are the roles of the following members of the multidisciplinary healthcare team members considering the nutritional needs of patients?

Team member	Roles
Registered nurse	Nurses carry out care on a 24-h basis as per instructions from other healthcare professionals. Nurses are essential for the delivery and evaluation of the prescribed care. Additionally, all other healthcare professionals will depend on the feedback received from nursing staff which will directly influence care delivery.
Doctor	To prescribe care as required for the patient in line with given anthropometric, biological and biochemical processes and subsequent results. Doctors also oversee the efficacy (or not) of interventions according to the results received and the patient's needs.
Healthcare assistant	Healthcare assistants are essential to the welfare of all patients as well as assisting the registered nurses in their role. Healthcare assistants are pivotal to essential care delivery and subsequent reporting and documentation of findings accordingly. Within their role, healthcare assistants can never be underestimated and their position within the multidisciplinary team is strengthening.
Dietician	Dieticians advise medical and nursing staff on the calorific content of certain diets with a view to ensuring that all patients have a well-balanced diet in line with their needs. Such a role includes suggesting appropriate dietary supplementary drinks which can be taken between meals to help boost a patient's appetite. Dieticians also observe the importance of biochemical results, especially magnesium and phosphorous levels. In addition to this, dieticians can set up feeding regimes when commencing enteral feeding via nasogastric tube, PEG tube or PEJ tube.
Speech and language therapist	Otherwise known as SALT, speech and language therapists are essential when assessing the safety of the patient's swallowing reflex. The swallowing reflex can be altered following neurological problems such as strokes, Parkinson's disease, motor neurone disease and multiple sclerosis. The results of the tests will yield information as to the consistency of the food which patients are allowed to eat safely. This information is documented in care notes and should be followed by all other healthcare professionals.
Nutrition coordinator	This job title usually falls under the remit of the ward housekeeper who carries out the ordering of foodstuffs and the distribution, completing and collection of menus on the ward. The nutrition coordinator usually coordinates the delivery of meals whilst testing the temperature of the said meals to prevent illness such as food poisoning. The nutrition coordinator also oversees the distribution of meals to the patients. He or she reports to the nursing staff about concerns regarding the lack of dietary intake by patients.

Activity 5.15

What issues do you think would need to be considered when looking at the practicalities of mealtimes within a hospital setting? Record your answers in the space provided.

Practicalities	Issues
Timing of meals	• Staff need to be aware of the timing of meals since the time lapse between breakfast and lunch may be only 3 h (0900 h and 1200 h). • Timing between supper (usually 1800 h) and breakfast the next morning (0900 h). • Are mealtimes occurring when there are visitors on the ward? Should protected mealtimes be strictly introduced, or should relatives be allowed to visit at mealtimes to assist with this important task? It is important that meals do not clash with other forms of therapy (e.g. physiotherapy or occupational therapy). If so, report this to the registered nurse.
Choice of meals	• Meals are usually taken from a pre-set menu which requires completion the previous day by the patient. • What happens if the patient does not understand language or different symbols on the menu? • What happens if the patient is moved from one clinical area to the other? • Many patients may not want three relatively large meal portions, but may want smaller and more frequent meal portions instead.
Where eating takes place	• Do the patients want to eat by their bedside? • Is there a dining room provided for the patients to eat their meals and, if so, is this dining room being used? • Is there enough space for the patient to manoeuvre for hand-to-mouth coordination?
Feeding utensils and other items such as condiments	• Are the eating utensils and implements appropriate for the patient in question?

(continued)

Activity 5.15 (*Continued*)

Practicalities	Issues
	• Does the patient have any neurological issues which may not allow the fine coordination of hand to mouth movements? • Are the implements being used appropriate for those with musculoskeletal disorders such as arthritis? • Do the utensils allow patients with limb weakness to feed himself or herself without food falling out over the sides? • Are condiments offered routinely and are restrictive dietary requirements taken into consideration? • Ensure that there are adequate fluids for the patients to drink with their meal.
Other issues	• Remember health and safety when giving out food and remember to use aprons and gloves as required. • If food comes in individual compartments with lids, please ensure that the lids are removed for those who cannot do so for themselves. • Be aware of any arrangements with the catering department should you have any patients attending other departments or hospitals for investigations. • Is your patient on oxygen therapy and wearing a face mask? If so, how will eating and drinking needs be met? Does the person need the oxygen mask or will nasal cannulae suffice for the delivery of the said oxygen therapy? • When patients are eating by their bedside and somebody needs the toilet, is the patient helped to the toilet or is a commode brought to the bedside for the patient to use? • Think of patients who are visibly impaired as they may not be able to see the food in front of them.

Activity 5.16

Reflect on your placement experience when you cared for patients with nutritional needs. Write in sentences what happened, how you felt and what would you do differently (if anything) next time when you care for someone with who required any assistance.

This is your personal experience of caring for patients who require assistance with their nutritional needs. Reflect your own personal feelings in relation to your learning needs. You may have more than one learning need; hence you could use the same subheadings to address the issues.

What happened?

- Describe the scenario briefly relating to your learning need.

How did it make you feel?

- Did you feel good or bad about it?
- What was good or bad about the situation?
- Did you have adequate underpinning knowledge to carry out the care?
- If you had previous experience of similar situation, was it useful this time?

What would you do differently (if anything) next time?

- Has this personal experience prepared you to do further reading and gained more practice under supervision?

This is only a guide. Please address the subheadings to meet your own learning needs.

References

Age Concern (2006) Hungry to be heard. In *The Scandal of Malnourished Older People in Hospital* (London: Age Concern England).

Alexander, M.F., Fawcett, J.N. and Runciman, P.J. (2006) *Nursing Practice Hospital & Home The Adult*, 3rd edn (Edinburgh: Churchill Livingstone).

Bennett, C. (2003) Assisting patients to meet their nutritional needs. In *Key Nursing Skills*, B.A. Workman and C.L. Bennett, eds (London: Whurr), pp. 214–234.

British Association for Parenteral and Enteral Nutrition (BAPEN) (2008) Malnutrition Universal Screening Tool (MUST). http://www.bapen.org.uk/must_tool.html (accessed 12 March 2008).

Brogden, B.J. (2004) Clinical skills: importance of nutrition for acutely ill hospital patients. *British Journal of Nursing* **13** (15), 914–920.

Department of Health (2001) *The Essence of Care* (London: Department of Health).

Department of Health (2008) Obesity General Information. www.dh.gov.uk/en/Publichealth/Healthimprovement/Obesity/DH_078098 (accessed 21 March 2008).

Dunne, A. (2007) Malnutrition: supplements and food fortification in the older population. *British Journal of Community Nursing* **12** (11), 494–499.

Green, S. and Jackson, P. (2006) Nutrition. In *Nursing Practice. Hospital and Home. The Adult*, 3rd edn, M.F. Alexander, J.N. Fawcett and P.J. Runciman, eds (Edinburgh: Churchill Livingstone Elsevier), pp. 787–812.

Green, S.M. and McLaren, S.G. (1998) Nutritional assessment and screening: instrument selection. *British Journal of Community Nursing* **3** (5), 233–242.

Grodner, M., Anderson, S. and DeYoung, S. (2000) *Foundations and Clinical Applications of Clinical Nutrition. A Nursing Approach*, 2nd edn (St. Louis: Mosby).

Hayward, J. (2003) Ward nutrition coordinators to improve patient nutrition in hospital. *British Journal of Nursing* **12** (18), 1081–1089.

Hearing, S. (2004) Refeeding syndrome. Is underdiagnosed and undertreated, but treatable. *British Medical Journal* **328** (7445), 908–909.

Heath, H. (ed.) (1995) *Potter and Perry's Foundations in Nursing Theory and Practice* (Philadelphia: Elsevier).

Hicks, R. (2005) Body Mass Index. http://www.bbc.co.uk/health/healthy_living/your_weight/bmiimperial_index.shtml (accessed 7 March 2008).

Isaac, M.T. and Isaac, M.B. (2004) *Eat Yourself Happy* (London: Carroll & Brown).

Kingsbury, S.D. (1999) The development of a policy for the administration of peripheral parenteral nutrition. *The Pharmaceutical Journal* **263** (7063), 46–47.

Kozier, B., Glenora, E., Berman, A., Snyder, S., Lake, R. and Harvey, S. (2008) *Fundamental of Nursing. Concepts, Process and Practice* (Harlow: Pearson Education).

Lennard-Jones, J. (1999) *Ethical and Legal Aspects of Fluid and Nutrients in Clinical Practice* (London: Nursing Times Books).

Martin, E. (ed.) (2003) *Oxford Dictionary of Nursing*, 4th edn (Oxford: Oxford University Press).

McFerran, T.A. and Maritn, E.A. (eds) (2003) *A Dictionary of Nursing*, 4th edn (Oxford: Oxford University Press).

McWhirter, J. and Pennington, C. (1994) Incidence and recognition of malnutrition in hospital. *British Medical Journal* **308** (6934), 945–948.

NHS Direct (2008a) Common health questions: what is the body mass index (BMI)? http://www.nhsdirect.nhs.uk/articles/article.aspx?articleId=850 (accessed 7 March 2008).

NHS Direct (2008b) Mind and body magazine: body mass index calculator. http://www.nhsdirect.nhs.uk/magazine/interactive/bmi/index.aspx# (accessed 7 March 2008).

National Institute for Health and Clinical Excellence (NICE) (2006) *Nutritional Support in Adults (Clinical Guideline 32)* (London: NICE).

National Patient Safety Agency (2005) Advice to the NHS on reducing harm caused by the misplacement of nasogastric feeding tubes. http://www.npsa.nhs.uk/patientsafety/alerts-and-directives/alerts/nasogastric-feeding-tubes/ (accessed 6 March 2008).

Nursing and Midwifery Council (2008) *The Code. Standards of Performance and Ethics for Nurses and Midwives* (London: NMC).

Pancorbo-Hidalgo, P.L., Garcia-Fernandez, F.P. and Ramirez-Perez, C. (2001) Complications associated with enteral nutrition by nasogastric tube in an internal medical unit. *Journal of Clinical Nursing* **10**, 482–490.

Porter, D. (2007) Countdown to zero. http://news.bbc.co.uk/1/hi/magazine/635077.stm (accessed 28 February 2008).

Roberts, E. (2007) Nutritional support via enteral tube feeding in hospital patients. *British Journal of Nursing* **16** (19), 1058–1062.

Say, J. (2005a) Eating and drinking: nutrient and fluid requirements for health. In *Compendium of Clinical Skills for Student Nurses*, I. Peate, ed. (London: Whurr), pp. 92–110.

Say, J. (2005b) Eating and drinking: nutrient and fluid replacement for health. In *Compendium of Clinical Skills for Student Nurses*, I. Peate, ed. (London: Whurr), pp. 111–137.

Selfe, L. (2006) Disorders of the urinary system. In *Nursing Practice. Hospital and Home. The Adult*, 3rd edn, M.F. Alexander, J.N. Fawcett and P.J. Runciman, eds (Edinburgh: Churchill Livingstone Elsevier), pp. 357–394.

Smith, A. (2008) Nutrition in care homes: back to basics. *Nursing and Residential Care* **10** (2), 68–72.

Walsh, M. (2003) Caring for a person with a disorder of the endocrine system. In *Watson's Clinical Nursing and Related Sciences*, 6th edn, M. Walsh, ed. (Edinburgh: Balliere Tindall), pp. 561–610.

Further reading

Alexander, M.F., Fawcett, J.N. and Runciman, P.J. (2006) *Nursing Practice Hospital & Home The Adult*, 3rd edn (Edinburgh: Churchill Livingstone).

British Association for Parenteral and Enteral Nutrition (BAPEN) (2008) *Malnutrition Universal Screening Tool (MUST)*. www.bapen.org.uk/must_tool.html.

Hayward, J. (2003) Ward nutrition coordinators to improve patient nutrition in hospital. *British Journal of Nursing* **12** (18), 1081–1089.

National Institute for Health and Clinical Excellence (NICE) (2006) *Nutritional Support in Adults (Clinical Guideline 32)* (London: NICE).

Roberts, E. (2007) Nutritional support via enteral tube feeding in hospital patients. *British Journal of Nursing* **16** (17), 1058–1062.

Sanders, D.S., Leeds, J. and Drew, K. (2008) The role of percutaneous endoscopic gastronomy in patients with dementia. *British Journal of Nursing* **17** (9), 588–594.

Seymour, S. (2000) Preoperative fluid restrictions: hospital policy and clinical practice. *British Journal of Nursing* **9** (14), 925–930.

Sinclair, J.M. (ed.) (2000) *The Times English Dictionary* (Glasgow: Market House Books).

Valentine, S. (2007) Nutrition for active kids. *British Journal of School Nursing* **2** (3), 122–126.

6 Principles of elimination

LOUISE LAWSON

Aims

The aim of this chapter is to introduce you to the key principles of elimination. It will provide an overview of urine and stool assessment and the care of patients who have toileting needs.

Learning objectives

On completion of this chapter, you will learn to:

- Recognise the principles of stool and urine observation with factors that affect bowel and urinary function
- Recognise predisposing factors leading to altered bowel habits
- Recognise predisposing factors leading to altered urinary habits
- Acknowledge the importance of privacy and dignity
- Outline the nursing management of toileting needs
- Understand the psychological impact of incontinence
- Distinguish normal and abnormal characteristics and composition of faeces and urine
- Complete the activities in order to prepare you for clinical placement and attendance of clinical skills sessions in relation to the elimination needs of your patient/client

Introduction

Elimination of urine and faeces is an essential bodily function that most of us perform without much thought and is a natural process critical for human functioning (Evans-Smith, 2005). However, elimination needs can become affected due to factors such as disability, physiological or psychological causes, which would then require assistance from you both in hospital or any other care setting. Being able to meet the needs of your patients both sensitively and professionally is an aspect of your work that is both essential and rewarding. Nursing interventions will be intimate and will require you to maintain privacy and dignity at all times, and to be able to gain trust and confidence due to the intimate nature of the care given. The 'skill' of assisting patients with elimination needs is noted in the Department of Health's document *Essence of Care* (DH, 2001) in which they outline 11 benchmarks for best practice. The document aimed to improve quality in care and was designed to share good practice.

Roper *et al.* (1990) describe eliminating as the excretion of waste products from the body which involves mainly the urinary and gastro-intestinal (GI) tract. This chapter will consider the anatomy and physiology of the GI and the urinary tract, with further reference to micturition and defaecation. This will help you to focus on the underpinning theory and will assist you in developing skills relating to bowel and urinary elimination in order to provide the necessary care for your patient. Discussion and activities will focus around your role as a student, assessment, management of care and health promotion. These will be apparent throughout the chapter, and will include communication, privacy and dignity of the patient and issues surrounding health and safety. This will provide you with a fundamental understanding of the essential core clinical skill of meeting elimination needs, thus supporting the development of professional competencies for your practice. This in turn aims to foster professional attributes necessary for you as students of healthcare to become effective learners in any practice environment in order to deliver safe, effective and competent care to your patients/clients (NMC, 2008). It is intended that this chapter will strengthen the development of skills whilst in your practice areas, or in a in a simulated environment.

In order for you to complete this chapter, you will need to do some revision of the anatomy and physiology of the urinary and GI system, paying particular attention to micturition and defaecation. Furthermore, think back to when you have cared for someone with elimination needs and try to draw on those experiences. These should help you when you are completing the activities. There are no right or wrong answers for some of the activities; these are about your experiences and how you apply them to your work; the answers to the activities however, can be found at the end of the chapter. You will also be required to review your local health policy regarding the disposal of excreta and infection control standards. These policies can be applied to both hospital and community settings. You may wish to discuss this chapter with your placement mentor or tutor.

Facing your fears

Caring for patients with elimination needs can often be daunting for the novice nurse. By identifying how this makes you feel may help you to be more confident and overcome any fears. Write in the shapes in Activity 6.1 some key words to describe how you feel when assisting patients with toileting needs.

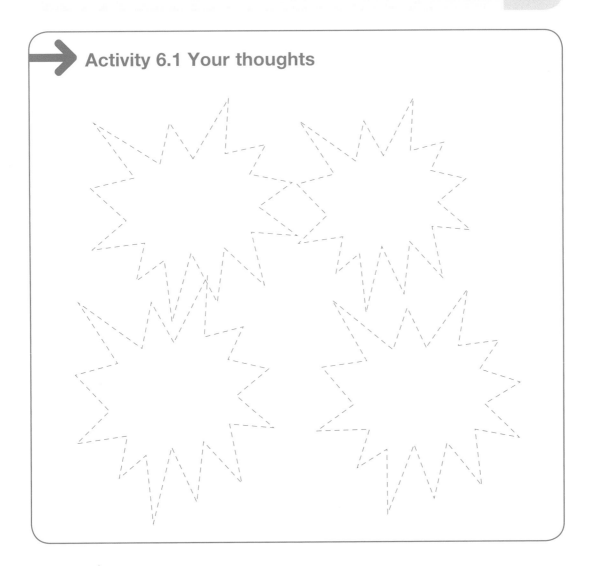

Activity 6.1 Your thoughts

Using your nursing dictionary, look up these words and write the definitions below:

Activity 6.2 Key terms

Nursing term	Definition
Colostomy	
Excretion	

(continued)

→ Activity 6.2 (*Continued*)

Nursing term	Definition
Melaena	
Constipation	
Ileostomy	
Enema	
Laxatives	
Flatulence	
Defaecation	
Diarrhoea	
Skatole	
Indole	
Some common prefixes	**Meaning**
Dys	
Pre	
Post	
Some common suffixes	
ostomy	
otomy	
ectomy	

Factors affecting elimination

Most people would have experienced some minor differences in their bowel movements, such as constipation and diarrhoea, and some people experience acute or chronic bowel problems affecting their fluid and electrolyte balance, hydration, nutritional status, skin integrity, comfort and self concept (Evans-Smith, 2005). This could be due to interventions such as surgery, diagnostic testing and illness; therefore, you play an essential role in the prevention, management and correction of any potential altered bowel habits. However, it could simply be embarrassment or reluctance to eliminate in an environment that is not familiar to them.

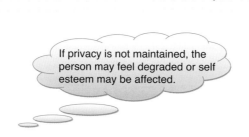

If privacy is not maintained, the person may feel degraded or self esteem may be affected.

There are many factors that affect elimination which could include physical, psychological, sociocultural, environmental and politico-economic (Pollard and Levy, 2005). Write down what you think these factors could be under the headings provided in Activity 6.3.

Activity 6.3 Factors affecting elimination

Physical factors	
Psychological factors	
Sociocultural factors	
Environmental factors	
Politics and economic factors	

Toileting amenities

In order to provide adequate toileting facilities for your patient, you need to identify any problems with elimination and then make an initial assessment on whether any assistance is required. You must work in partnership with your patients and be able to assess which is the most appropriate vessel for them to eliminate into based on their physical or emotional ability. Whenever possible, try to offer your patient the toilet which is more familiar to everyone and ultimately maintains the most privacy. This not only promotes psychological well-being, but also maintains normality despite ill health or disability (Hilton, 2004) and can be achieved by assisting the patient walking to the toilet, or onto a commode and wheeling to the bathroom. Certain adaptations can be made to the toilet if required, such as raised toilet seat or handrails.

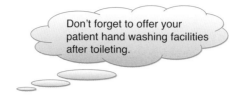

Don't forget to offer your patient hand washing facilities after toileting.

The commode Figure 6.1) can also be used inside the curtains around the bed; however, be aware that this may not feel very private for the patient as noises can be heard and smells more apparent. This potential embarrassment could lead the patient ignoring the need to defaecate, which could lead to constipation (Edwards, 1997).

Remember; maintain safety by not leaving frail or vulnerable patients alone on a commode by the bedside.

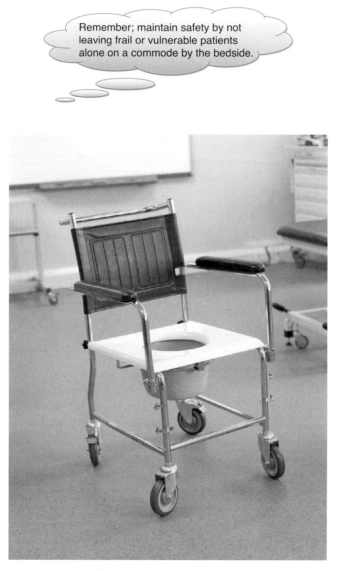

Figure 6.1   A commode

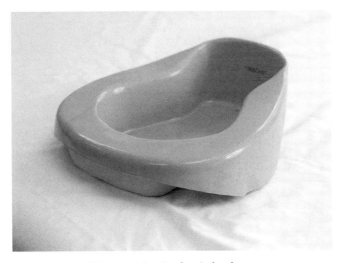

Figure 6.2   A plastic bedpan

Tarling (1997) discusses types of commodes and their advantages and disadvantages with particular reference to moving and handling. Patients who cannot get out of bed however, will need assistance to pass urine or have their bowels open. You will need to assess the limitations of your patients and their ability to use variances in appliances such as a urinal, or a bedpan (see Figure 6.2). Again, you need to make an assessment of the patient's needs and choose between a slipper bedpan of which the patient can roll onto, or the standard bedpan which can be sat on whilst in bed. A urinal can be used for a male whose mobility is limited and can be used in bed or whilst sitting on the edge of the bed. Most bedpans and urinals are disposable these days; however, if in an alternative placement, you may need to rinse out the receptacle under the hot water tap, though this does not affectively disinfect as the ideal temperature needs to reach 25°C (Baillie, 2001). However, Ayliffe *et al.* (1999) recommend disinfection of non-disposable bedpans and urinals by heat. Remember to wash your hands and offer hand-washing facilities to your patient.

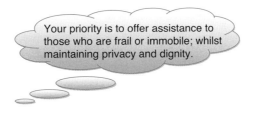

Your priority is to offer assistance to those who are frail or immobile; whilst maintaining privacy and dignity.

Reflection point
Think of examples of patients you may have cared for who have required assistance with toileting.

Activity 6.4 Patients who need help

Write down some of the reasons why they may have needed your help.

There are many items of equipment that can assist you when helping a patient with toileting needs. Briefly describe the purpose of these items of equipment below:

Activity 6.5 Equipment

Equipment	Purpose
Commode	
Urinal	
Bedpan	

Be aware of how frightening sitting on a commode may be to some as well as being uncomfortable after long periods.

Activity 6.6 Appropriate vessel

Which would be the most appropriate vessel for an elderly lady who has recently had spinal surgery?

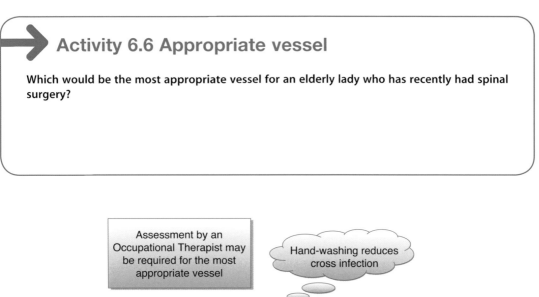

Assessment by an Occupational Therapist may be required for the most appropriate vessel

Hand-washing reduces cross infection

Remember to leave your patient with a replacement urinal so they do not have to wait for another one.

Privacy and dignity

The RCN (2008) believe that dignity is fundamental in all care and that nurses should prioritise dignity in care, placing it at the heart of all we do. The definition of dignity incorporates many of the characteristics of privacy of the person: respect for the person, privacy of the body, privacy of one's space and territory, and having control and choice of one's surroundings (Walsh and Kowanko, 2002; Woogara, 2004). When patients are not feeling well, they would like you to help them to rest and provide comfort and be able to ensure that their privacy and dignity is maintained. Patients have a right to privacy and dignity (DH, 2001) which should be respected at all times. These rights are highlighted in the Human Rights Act (1998), which enables the incorporation of the European Convention of Human Rights in UK legislation. Following the passing of this law, a number of Department of Health (DH) publications (DH, 2000, 2001) have emphasised the importance of healthcare practitioners respecting the privacy and dignity of patients in NHS care settings. It is your role to uphold privacy and dignity, and this can be achieved in many ways. Check out factors 6 and 7 in the seven factors relating to privacy and dignity in the document *Essence of Care* (DH, 2001) and read how you can actively promote privacy, dignity and modesty for your patients.

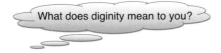

What does dignity mean to you?

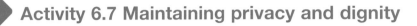

Activity 6.7 Maintaining privacy and dignity

Briefly describe what steps you would take to maintain privacy, dignity and modesty when giving a commode or bedpan?

Health and safety issues

When assisting a patient with elimination, it is important to consider how you would prevent the transmission of infection. The danger of cross-infection in a clinical environment is increased, but can be minimised by recognising steps to reduce any risk. Evidence indicates that improvements in infection control practice can reduce the incidence of healthcare-associated infection and exposure to communicable disease among healthcare workers and patients (Tenorio *et al.*, 2001; Flores, 2007). Patients who are unwell are particularly vulnerable to infection and are at potentially high-risk of infection; therefore, you are the key person in the prevention of cross-infection by key elements, such as washing your hands, correct disposal of equipment and safe management of spillages and accidents. By washing your hands effectively you can contribute to the eradication of transmission of infection between your patients, visitors and their families. Your clinical area will have produced infection control policies and guidelines for staff when caring for patients. These must be adhered to, so have a look at the policies next time when caring for patients. Also, look at some of the posters on your placement and see how they demonstrate effective handwashing. You must remember to wash your hands before and after contact with the patient and again if your hands are soiled.

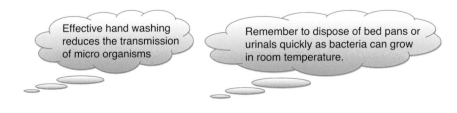

Effective hand washing reduces the transmission of micro organisms

Remember to dispose of bed pans or urinals quickly as bacteria can grow in room temperature.

> **Activity 6.8 Factors to consider**
>
> What factors would you consider before and after a patient has used the toilet, or have been in contact with bodily fluids?

Communication

Eliminating is a very private activity, and your attitude and non-verbal body language can affect the patient in the future when asking to use the toilet. Patients should at all times be given the choice of how they would like to go to the toilet, for example a bedpan, a commode or to be escorted to the toilet. Remember, if you leave a patient on a commode or bedpan, remember to leave a call bell and come back to check on his or her progress. Communication is an integral part of the nurse's role. The essential skills clusters (NMC, 2007) relate to the outcomes and proficiencies in The Code (NMC, 2008) and the Standards of Proficiency for Pre-registration Nursing Education (NMC, 2004) highlight the importance of communication skills and why effective communication is so crucial to nursing practice. You must communicate with your patient in a way that indicates that his or her individuality, personal identity and dignity are respected and not compromise your relationship by failing to do so. To ensure effective communication, you must start with an assessment of the patients' ability to understand and their use of non-verbal cues, for instance facial expression. Before you complete the activities, reflect back on your experiences whilst on clinical placement and use these experiences to complete the activity below.

> **Activity 6.9 Communication skills**
>
> What communication skills would you use when caring for a patient with elimination needs?

The topic of elimination may be embarrassing for the patient or even you to discuss, although it is a significant part of nursing care. Many patients are too embarrassed to discuss bowel function and will often delay in reporting problems despite the impact the symptoms have on their quality of life (Cadd et al., 2000). Effective communication can help to alleviate stress and anxiety when being toileted and sensitivity is required in order to dispel embarrassment and ensure a shared understanding of the meaning of the terms used by the patient (Smith, 2001). Women with multiple sclerosis have spoken of feelings of 'humiliation' at having to ask for help with elimination (Koch and Kelly, 1999), and if you do not appear approachable, patients may feel that they cannot ask for your help.

Activity 6.10 Barriers to communication

What barriers to communication could cause elimination problems?

Be aware of non-verbal cues/communication such as restlessness, body language and facial expressions.

Write in the activity below some common words people use for going to the toilet.

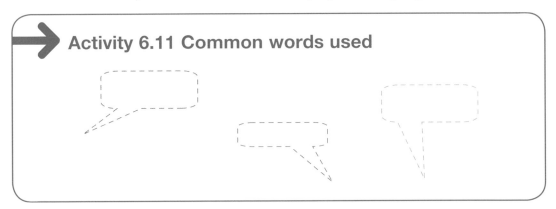

Activity 6.11 Common words used

Bowel elimination

This section will look specifically at bowel elimination and will discuss the anatomy and physiology of the alimentary tract. It will cover the skills required to assist patients with constipation, diarrhoea and the assessment and management of both. This section will also enable you to promote and assist others with bowel elimination as many patients may experience different factors that affect their bowel function whilst in hospital. This could be due to diagnostic testing, poor diet or surgical interventions. Therefore, you as a healthcare professional play an integral role in the promotion, education and prevention of disease, and management of bowel elimination.

Anatomy and physiology

An understanding of bowel function is necessary in order for you to be able to undertake an assessment. The alimentary tract is a continuous tract and is approximately 10 m long from the mouth to the anus (Nair, 2005). It is also known as the gastro-intestinal tract (GI) or the digestive tract. The main functions of the GI tract are ingestion, digestion, absorption and excretion. The small bowel is approx 6.4 m in length (Mader, 1997) and divided into three sections: the duodenum, jejunum and ileum. The bowel provides a large surface for absorption and digestion and the contents are moved along the length of the bowel by peristalsis, which means that the food is passed along the bowel by rhythmic contractions of smooth muscles. Digestion and absorption occur in the small intestine which begins at the pyloric sphincter of the stomach; it coils around the abdomen and opens into the large intestine at the ileocaecal junction (Dougherty and Lister, 2008).

Peristalsis happens around 3 to 4 times per day which begins at the middle of the transverse colon and then drives the contents of the bowel into the rectum for excretion. The large bowel or the colon is approximately 1.5 m in length and its main function is to store faeces. It eliminates the waste products of digestion and produces mucous to lubricate the faecal mass. It also absorbs fluids, electrolytes and synthesises vitamins B and K and secretes many digestive enzymes by the small intestine (Tortora and Grabowski, 2002). Seventy percent of food is excreted within 72 h (Bisanz, 2007) and the remaining 30% may remain in the bowel for up to a week or more. The longer the faeces remain in the bowel, the more water is absorbed, which can be up to 2 L of water in 24 h (Dougherty and Lister, 2008), the harder the faeces become. This then makes it difficult to pass thus experiencing constipation.

Label the diagram of the main components of the digestive system.

Activity 6.12

The key words are to help you to complete the diagram. Now identify the function of each component of the digestive tract.

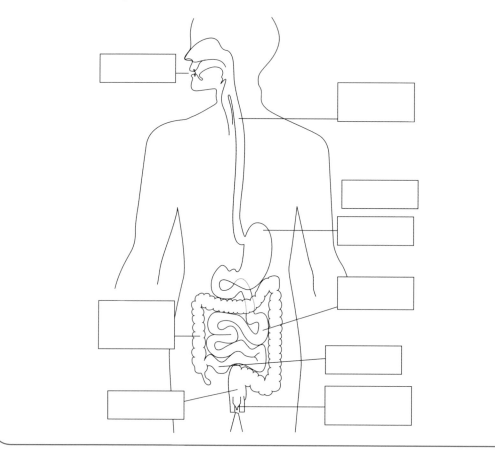

Activity 6.13 Key words

Key word	Function
Mouth	
Oesophagus	

Activity 6.13 (*Continued*)

Stomach	
Large intestine	
Small intestine	
Rectum	
The anal canal	

Defaecation is the expulsion of faeces from the anus and rectum and is also called a bowel movement (Kozier *et al.*, 2004). A stool should look brown in colour, be formed, semisolid and eliminated everyday; however, this can vary from person to person depending on his or her diet and other factors.

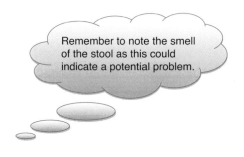

Remember to note the smell of the stool as this could indicate a potential problem.

Activity 6.14 What your stool should look like?

Write down what your stool looked liked the last time you had your bowels open.

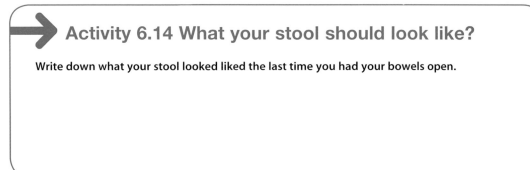

Diet is clearly an important factor in bowel management. If the stool is too hard, a fibre supplement might be required. Alternatively if the stool is too soft, it may be more sensible to reduce the fibre intake. The promotion of a healthy diet is integral to optimum health, independence and quality of life and is an integral component of overall health, independence and quality of life in older people (Neno and Neno, 2006). Food entering the body must be broken down and absorbed if it is to be used positively (Marieb, 2004). It is essential that you are aware of the sociological, biological and economic factors that affect the ability for people to consume a healthy diet, particularly in later life.

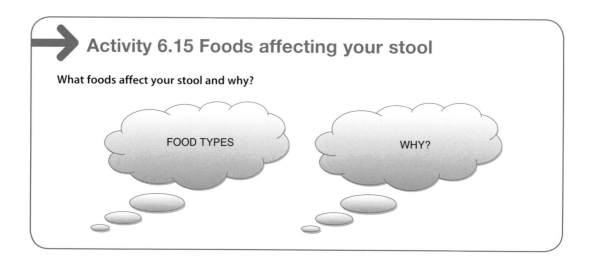

Activity 6.15 Foods affecting your stool

What foods affect your stool and why?

FOOD TYPES

WHY?

Activity 6.16 Constituents of stool

Write here what you think your stool consists of.

Accurate evaluation and documentation of the care that you give is a professional requirement. The Nursing and Midwifery Code states that 'you must ensure that the healthcare record for the patient or client is an accurate account of treatment, care planning and delivery' (Nursing and Midwifery Council: The Code, 2008). You may also wish to read the *Guidelines for Records and Record Keeping* (Nursing and Midwifery Council, 2005). When observing faeces, you should note any abnormalities and document your findings accurately and immediately after you have made your assessment.

➡️ **Activity 6.17 Factors to consider**

Write down what you should consider when observing your patient's stool.

This section will focus on the risk factors and assessment for constipation and diarrhoea and will discuss some issues which help to prevent and manage these conditions. It is generally accepted that the passing of at least three stools per week, without straining, may be considered as normal; however, three times per day can also be considered normal for others (Bisanz, 2007), depending on factors such as how much food is consumed, any medication taken and the amount of fluid or fibre ingested.

Constipation

Constipation is characterised by infrequent, hard dry stools which may be difficult to pass. One useful definition is that constipation is the passage of hard stools less frequently than the patient's own normal pattern (British National Formulary, 2006) and usually accompanied by excessive straining (Barrett, 2002). However, there appears to be much debate about what constitutes a clear definition of constipation (Richmond, 2003), and these are open to many variances which can often lead to confusion. The patient may complain of a feeling of incomplete emptying of the rectum which then becomes enlarged causing pain and discomfort. Constipation may occur due to the slowing down of the contents through to the large intestine and decrease of the contractions of the rectum when filled with stool (Kauffman, 1999). In assessing bowel dysfunction, it is important to establish what has been the client's usual bowel function in the past. This is to clarify what has been 'normal' for them. Abnormal bowel movements can be very distressing for your patients, so assessment is very important when managing patients. For the successful management of constipation, this requires you to discover the underlying causes and discuss ways of preventing reoccurrence.

➡️ **Activity 6.18 Predisposing factors causing constipation**

Write down the possible causes why a patient could suffer from constipation.

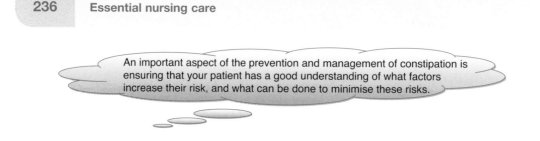

An important aspect of the prevention and management of constipation is ensuring that your patient has a good understanding of what factors increase their risk, and what can be done to minimise these risks.

Assessment of stool

A bowel assessment chart should be completed by the patient/carer. The use of Bristol Stool Chart (Gill, 1999) is universally accepted. A stool may consist of one or more types.

The Bristol Stool Chart in Figure 6.3 can be used to define stool types. Types 3–4 are generally considered to be 'normal' stool consistency. The colour and consistency of faecal matter can provide important information to assist diagnosis and to monitor your patient's condition.

Another bowel assessment chart is the Kings Stool Chart (2001) which can be freely downloaded from www.kcl.ac.uk/stoolchart

Activity 6.19 Prevention of constipation

What factors would you consider when giving information to a patient in the prevention of constipation?

Education and advice on diet and fluid intake should be the first step in the management of all constipated patients.

THE BRISTOL STOOL FORM SCALE

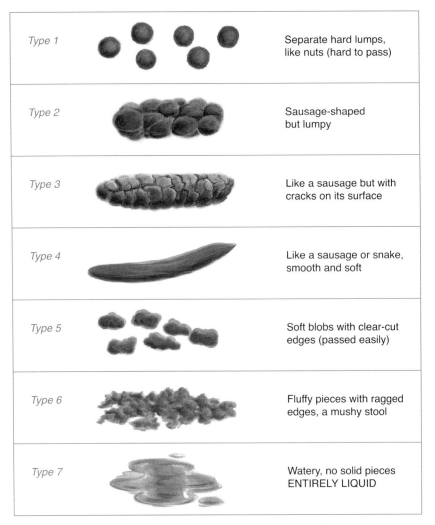

Type 1		Separate hard lumps, like nuts (hard to pass)
Type 2		Sausage-shaped but lumpy
Type 3		Like a sausage but with cracks on its surface
Type 4		Like a sausage or snake, smooth and soft
Type 5		Soft blobs with clear-cut edges (passed easily)
Type 6		Fluffy pieces with ragged edges, a mushy stool
Type 7		Watery, no solid pieces ENTIRELY LIQUID

Figure 6.3   The Bristol Stool Chart, reproduced with permission

Treatment and management

Prodigy Guidance (2008) advises a stepped approach to the management of constipation. This topic review undertaken by the National Health Service (NHS) has reviewed the management of constipation in detail and made recommendations which are more clearly justified and transparently linked to the supporting evidence. This review offers clearer advice on treatment strategies, more detail on the advantages and disadvantages of the different laxatives and more detail on foods and diets that may be useful in managing constipation. The Prodigy Guidance (2008) recommends that if the response to oral laxatives is insufficient or not fast enough,

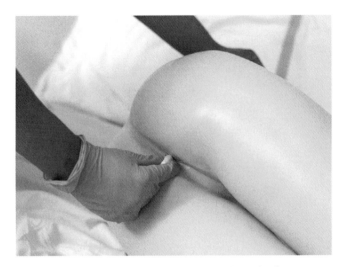

Figure 6.4   Inserting a suppository into the bottom

consider using a suppository such as bisacodyl for soft stools; glycerol alone or glycerol plus bisacodyl for hard stools. Suppositories can be administered as a treatment for constipation or can be given to administer medication, such as a local treatment for haemorrhoids. They should not be administered for chronic constipation or any evidence of bowel obstruction and will need to be prescribed. Glycerine suppositories can act as a rectal stimulant due to the mild irritant action of glycerol (RPS and BMA, 2008). These should be lubricated before insertion and patient will need to lie on his or her left side in order to insert the suppository correctly (see Figure 6.4). The suppository must be placed alongside the bowel wall, as if placed directly into the faeces; the heat of the body cannot melt the glycerol so serves no purpose (Kyle, 2006). There is much confusion in relation to the correct method for insertion of suppositories which stems from a study in the *Lancet* by Abd-El-Maeboud *et al.* (1991) who stated that suppositories should be inserted blunt end first. This is, however, contested in a paper written by Bradshaw and Price (2007) who conclude that it is clear that there is little reliable evidence for supporting the method of blunt end foremost as opposed to what is described as the 'commonsense' method of pointed end foremost. It is important to read the manufactures' instructions before inserting a suppository, and to look at the policies and practice in your clinical area to see which method is used.

Think about patients who have a physical disability and how this may affect their bowel habits.

Activity 6.20 Position of patient

What position would you place a patient before administering a suppository and why?

Activity 6.21 Advice to patient

What advice would you give to your patient after administering a suppository?

Diarrhoea

Disorders of bowel function resulting in diarrhoea are not unusual and chronic diarrhoea is one of the most common causes of hospital admission (Thomas *et al.*, 2003). Diarrhoea can be defined as an abnormal increase in the quantity, frequency and fluid content of stool and is associated with urgency, perineal discomfort and incontinence (Bashe, 1987). This occurs when the imbalance among absorption, secretion and intestinal motility is disturbed (Hogan, 1998). Diarrhoea is a symptom and can be acute, which is usually caused by a viral or bacterial infection and can affect almost everyone at some time in their lives. It is usually accompanied by stomach pains, nausea and vomiting. Chronic diarrhoea is normally caused by a disorder of the alimentary tract and will need to be investigated. Remember to consider the patients' hygiene needs and skin care when they are suffering from chronic diarrhoea; however, this needs to be approached in a sensitive manner as some patients may be offended by the suggestion that they need to improve their personal hygiene (Norton, 2006). Furthermore, privacy and dignity must be maintained at all times.

Activity 6.22 Observation of stool

Write down what you would observe for when a patient experiences a bout of acute diarrhoea.

Activity 6.23 Causes of diarrhoea

List some disorders that could cause chronic diarrhoea.

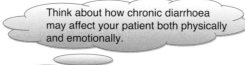

Think about how chronic diarrhoea
may affect your patient both physically
and emotionally.

Activity 6.24 Nursing care

What nursing care would be required for a patient suffering from chronic diarrhoea?

Before reading the next section, reflect on any assessments you have carried out on patients with bowel dysfunction. What vital signs did you record? Where did you record these observations? What implications do these have for your nursing practice?

Your reflections here…

This aspect of the chapter will focus on urinary needs, including activities relating to the urinary system, urinary tract infection (UTI) and urinalysis.

Urinary needs

Elimination through the urinary tract is a normal process of eliminating waste from the body. People can usually feel when their bladder is full and will then go on to empty their bladder in their usual way. Control of urinary elimination is usually developed by the age of 6 years (Carr, 1996); however, there can be many factors that affect the volume, characteristics and control of urinary elimination, whatever the age, such as disability, physiological and psychological factors. Many medications can impact on the passing of urine, particularly those affecting the autonomic nervous system, which interfere with the normal urination process and may cause retention (Kozier *et al.*, 2008). Many conditions can make people unable to feel bladder fullness, or can cause loss of control over urination. People with brain or spinal cord injuries, for example, may not be able to control the emptying of their bladder. Also, older people who are confused or suffer from dementia may not know when their bladder is full or cannot control the muscles used to urinate; however, if their muscles are functioning, they can voluntarily control urination. Most adults' urinary patterns are highly individual, though most pass around 1500 mL of urine five times per day (Kozier *et al.*, 2008). Managing urinary needs is a key element of your role as a healthcare professional. Nurses need to be sensitive, empathetic and use effective communication skills to help people with elimination problems (Baillie and Arrowsmith, 2005).

The urinary system

You will need to have an understanding of normal physiology of the urinary tract as well as associated factors that can cause potential renal problems. The principal function of the urinary system is to maintain the volume and composition of body fluids within normal limits. One aspect of this function is to rid the body of waste products that accumulate as a result of cellular metabolism and because of this, it is sometimes referred to as the excretory system (Selfe, 2006).

Although the urinary system has a major role in excretion, other organs contribute to the excretory function. The urinary system maintains an appropriate fluid volume by regulating the amount of water that is excreted in the urine. Other aspects of its function include regulating the concentrations of various electrolytes in the body fluids and maintaining normal pH of the blood (Edwards, 2001). In addition to maintaining fluid homeostasis in the body, the urinary system controls red blood cell production by secreting the hormone erythropoietin (Flanning, 2000). The urinary system also plays a role in maintaining normal blood pressure by secreting the enzyme rennin (Steggall (2007b).

The urinary system consists of two kidneys, two ureters, a bladder and a urethra. The two kidneys are responsible for water and electrolyte balance and the formation of urine by simple filtration, selective reabsorption and secretion (Pollard and Levy, 2005). The functional unit of the kidney is called the nephron; each kidney contains 1 million nephrons, and each nephron consists of a vascular and a tubular system (Henke and Eigsti, 2003). The kidneys produce urine by filtering blood, which is then channelled into the bladder by the ureters (Marieb, 2004). When the bladder is full (approx. 200–400 mL in adults), urine is then expelled from the bladder into the urethra and out of the body. In men, the urethra is approximately 25 cm long, curved and passes through the prostate gland which lies under the bladder; in women, the urethra is much shorter, straight and approximately 10 cm in length (Steggall, 2007b).

Activity 6.25

List here the functions of the kidney.

Micturition, voiding and urination/urinating are words you may hear for emptying the bladder.

Activity 6.26 The urinary system

Label the diagram of the urinary tract. The key words are here to help you to complete the diagram.

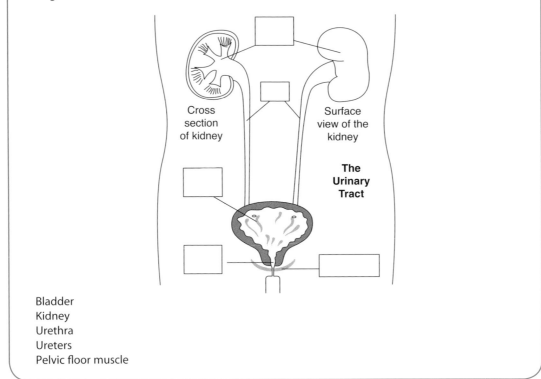

Cross section of kidney

Surface view of the kidney

The Urinary Tract

Bladder
Kidney
Urethra
Ureters
Pelvic floor muscle

Overview of the urinary system

- The urinary system rids the body of waste materials, regulates fluid volume, maintains electrolyte concentrations in body fluids, controls blood pH, secretes erythropoietin and rennin.
- The urinary system is made up of two kidneys, two ureters, a urinary bladder and a urethra.
- The cortex and medulla are the main parts of the kidney.
- The central region of the kidney is the renal pelvis, which collects the urine as it is produced.
- The functional unit of the kidney is a nephron, which consists of a renal corpuscle and a renal tubule.
- The ureters transport urine from the kidney to the urinary bladder.
- The urinary bladder is a temporary storage reservoir for urine.
- The urethra is the final passageway for the flow of urine.
- The flow of urine through the urethra is controlled by an involuntary internal urethral sphincter and voluntary external urethral sphincter.

Activity 6.27 Key terms

Now identify the meaning of each of these words.

Key term	Definition
Haematuria	
Glycosuria	
Micturition	
Ketonuria	
Proteinuria	
Anuria	
Dysuria	
Oliguria	
Polyuria or diuresis	
Acute urinary retention	

Urine infection

The Health Protection Agency (HPA, 2005) defines a UTI as the presence and multiplication of bacteria in one or more structures of the urinary tract. UTIs are a common problem in healthcare, and account for 1–3% of consultations in primary care (Hill, 2006). Urinary infections can affect people of all ages and is one of the most common bacterial infections resulting in pyrexia in children under the age of 2 years (Naish and Hallam, 2007). The incidence of men having a UTI increases with age and is often attributed to physiological changes associated with the aging process (Sinclair and Woodhouse, 1995); so it is important for you to understand how to care for people who have a UTI. Multiple factors can contribute to a UTI. Women are especially susceptible to bacteria which may invade the urinary tract and multiply resulting in infection. Though painful, these infections can easily treated with antibiotics which cause the symptoms to quickly disappear.

The most common cause of a UTI is bacteria from the bowel that live on the skin near the rectum or in the vagina which can spread and enter the urinary tract through the urethra. Once these bacteria enter the urethra, they travel upwards causing infection in the bladder and sometimes other parts of the urinary tract. Sexual intercourse can be a common cause of UTIs because the female anatomy can make women more prone to UTIs.

Activity 6.28

What else do you think can cause UTI?

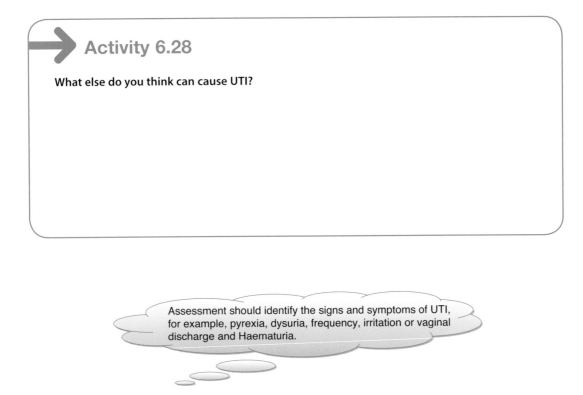

Assessment should identify the signs and symptoms of UTI, for example, pyrexia, dysuria, frequency, irritation or vaginal discharge and Haematuria.

Think about any patients you may have nursed who may have had a UTI and have a go at the activities below:

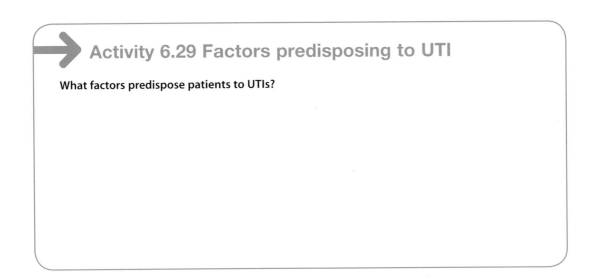

Activity 6.29 Factors predisposing to UTI

What factors predispose patients to UTIs?

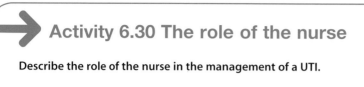

Activity 6.30 The role of the nurse

Describe the role of the nurse in the management of a UTI.

Urinalysis

Urinalysis is the testing of urine for a variety of substances, which will give valuable and immediate information about your patient's kidneys, urinary tract and liver, and will often influence the patient's subsequent management (Rowell, 1998). Urinalysis is also an important part of patient assessment and could potentially indicate the presence of serious disease (Steggall, 2007a).

A complete assessment of the patient's urinary function is crucial and is vital to the management of care. You can do this by using reagent strips which are easy to use and are a quick way of monitoring disease and identifying new illness. The strips are usually stored in a cupboard in the sluice room. Reagent strips are cost effective and reduce the need for laboratory testing (McGhee, 2004).

Next time you are in the practice area, find the reagent strips and note the colours on the strip and what they are tested for. Consider the significance of pH and specific gravity.

> Make sure reagent strips are in date as this could affect the result

Testing your patient's urine is an essential component of patient assessment which is used for screening, diagnosis and planning care (Wilson, 2005). Symptoms of UTIs are a common reason for seeking medical advice and are often overdiagnosed and overtreated; however, these have potential to cause serious complications, such as renal failure, if untreated (Sander, 2007). Healthcare professionals are often the first to detect a UTI by testing a person's urine. For example, the estimated number of undiagnosed persons with diabetes mellitus in England is 1 million (Chiasson et al., 2003) and without treatment, people are at higher risk of developing complications of this condition, such as hypertension, renal dysfunction, neuropathy and sexual dysfunction. It is also imperative that you maintain privacy and dignity and eliminate embarrassment when a urine sample is requested from your patient. You can do this by ensuring that curtains are drawn around the bed or the toilet door is closed before a sample is taken.

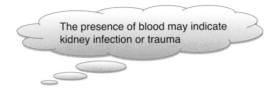

The presence of blood may indicate kidney infection or trauma

➡️ Activity 6.31 Urinalysis and its purpose

Describe in your own words what urinalysis is and the purpose of this assessment?

In order to take a urine sample, you will need to inform the patient and gain consent. The patient should be able enough to void into the toilet or a bedpan to produce a mid stream urine sample (MSU), or a sample can be collected from a catheter-specimen of urine (CSU). Most adults pass on average 200–400 mL of urine; however, around 50 mL is enough for a sample and patients are asked to catch a middle part of the void where possible (Smith *et al.*, 2004). Once the sample has been produced, it is sent to the laboratory usually for microscopy, culture and sensitivity to identify the presence of infection and the most effective treatment.

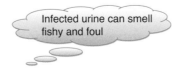

Infected urine can smell fishy and foul

Activity 6.32 Component of urine

What do you think the main component of urine is and what should a normal specimen look like?

Always use a fresh sample of urine for testing

Activity 6.33 Factors that affect urine output

What factors may increase or decrease urine output?

Activity 6.34 Glycosuria

What is the commonest cause of glucose found in a patient's urine?

Activity 6.35 Reflection

Reflect on your placement experiences when dealing with elimination needs of a patient. Write in sentences what happened, how did it make you feel and what would you do differently (if anything) next time when the patient requires assistance with elimination.

What happened?

How did it make you feel?

What would you do differently (if anything) next time?

Case Studies: Consider the case studies below and discuss some of the issues with your mentor or supervisor at work.

Case study 6.1

Mrs Jones, aged 89, has been admitted to the medical ward with chronic constipation. She lives alone in a warden controlled home and receives meals on wheels once per day. She is mobile but requires a Zimmer frame to assist in her walking. She is in considerable pain from her arthritic hip and has not had her bowels open for 7 days. She has been prescribed lactulose twice daily and two suppositories immediately. She admits that she does not drink enough fluids nor eat enough fruit and fibre foods.

Consider the care that you would give to this lady and what advice would you give her before she goes home, to prevent this from reoccurring? You can discuss this with your mentor or a nurse that you work with whilst in the clinical area.

Case study 6.2

Emily, aged 22, was presented in the emergency department with pain on micturition, passing blood in her urine and a strong urge to urinate frequently. She is pyrexial and complains of pain in her abdomen and back. She admits to having several sexual partners recently and uses the contraceptive pill only for contraception. Consider what may be wrong with her and why this may be the case. What actions would you take to care for this young lady and what advice could you give to her before discharge to prevent this from reoccurring? You can discuss this with your mentor or a nurse that you work with whilst in the clinical area.

Chapter summary

The management of elimination can be awkward and uncomfortable for you and your patient. Often, if you or your patient is embarrassed, professionalism and patience is invaluable. Furthermore, remember to involve your patients in any treatment or management of elimination, which will make them feel that they are not alone and have some control over their care. Successful management depends on good assessment and good assessment depends on your understanding of how the body works and why sometimes things can go wrong. You may need to involve other members of the inter-professional team who have specific expertise in this area and can be invaluable in assisting you with your learning. This chapter has provided an overview of toileting needs and the management of constipation, diarrhoea and urinary needs. The content of this chapter is by no means exhaustive as there is much more to be discussed, such as other treatments for constipation, catheter care and much more. You should now be able to understand why it is important to develop a culture that maintains privacy and dignity and uphold health and safety for all whom you care for. You have attempted activities relating to the elimination of stool and urine, including assessment and management of toileting, urinalysis and stool. These should begin to provide you with the knowledge and skills to assist or care for patients with elimination needs. You will also begin to build on your assessment skills which will enable you to develop as a healthcare professional and provide you with an opportunity to provide education and engage with your patients.

Answers to Activities

Activity 6.1 Your thoughts

These are your thoughts and personal to you. However, fear and anxiety can be overcome by knowledge and experience. Practice makes perfect and applying underpinning knowledge strengthens confidence and develops competence.

Activity 6.2 key terms

Nursing term	Definition
Colostomy	Artificial opening that permits faeces from the colon to exit through a stoma
Excretion	It is the process of eliminating waste products of metabolism and other non-useful materials
Melaena	Blood in stool could indicate upper gastric bleed. Could indicate malignancy
Constipation	Passage of hard, dry stools
Ileostomy	Artificial opening created to allow liquid faecal content from the ileum to be eliminated from the stoma
Enema	Introduction of a solution into the large intestine via the anus
Laxatives	Drugs to induce bowel movement. Can be oral or suppositories
Flatulence	The presence of intestinal gas (wind)
Defaecation	Emptying of the large intestine, also called a bowel movement
Diarrhoea	Passage of excessively liquid, non-formed stool
Skatole	A white, crystalline, water-soluble solid, found naturally in faeces
Indole	A colourless to yellow solid found in faeces
Some common prefixes	**Meaning**
Dys	Difficulty
Pre	Before
Post	After
Some common suffixes	
ostomy	Creation of an opening
otomy	Cutting into
ectomy	Surgical removal of

Activity 6.3 Factors affecting elimination

Physical factors	This could be an alteration in the structure, function or processes of the urinary, gastro-intestinal or associated bodily systems
Psychological factors	This could include intellect, anxiety and stress
Sociocultural factors	Patients use different words for elimination, different rituals surrounding elimination (such as clean hand for eating/dirty hand for cleansing), fasting and other dietary restrictions
Environmental factors	This could include poor storage of food, poor personal hygiene and poor toileting facilities
Politics and economic factors	This could be due to lack of finances for a healthy high-fibre diet, political influences on availability of foods (Hilton, 2004)

Activity 6.4 Patients who need help

Write down some of the reasons why they may have needed your help.
You may have considered conditions such as patients who are temporarily confined to bed following major surgery, a patient who is breathless, spinal or neurological conditions or just someone who is frail, generally unwell or on bed rest.

Activity 6.5 Equipment

Equipment	Purpose
Commode	If your patient is able to get out of bed, then a commode is preferable as this can be wheeled to the toilet or used at the bedside with a bedpan underneath.
Urinal	Used for males and can be used in bed or at the bedside. Can also be disposable.
Bedpan	This can be a standard shape or flat slipper and are mainly disposable. If macerators are not available, the contents can be disposed in the toilet and washed with soap and water. Bedpans for male and female are often available.

Activity 6.6 Appropriate vessel

Which would be the most appropriate vessel for an elderly lady who has recently had spinal surgery?
A flat slipper bedpan would be best for someone who has had spinal surgery, as they can roll onto the pan if they cannot sit up.

Activity 6.7 Maintaining privacy and dignity

Briefly describe what steps you would take to maintain privacy, dignity and modesty when giving a commode or bedpan?
When thinking about maintaining privacy and dignity in relation to toileting, you would consider factors such as drawing curtains around the bed and ensuring that they are properly shut, or the toilet door is closed properly. Ensure that urinals are removed immediately from the bedside and never leave lying around to do later. You would also consider covering a patient when using the bedpan or commode and being sensitive to people's non-verbal cues. It is important that you are aware of cultural differences and do not make any assumptions. You should speak quietly and privately when assisting a patient with elimination. All UK citizens have legal, ethical, expected and human rights when they are admitted to NHS hospitals (Woogara, 2004). The publication of the *Essence of Care* (DH, 2001) was designed to improve the quality of care and strengthen the notion that privacy of the person is important. The document also identifies seven factors relating to privacy and dignity against which healthcare professionals should benchmark their practice. This document can be found on www.dh.gov.uk and search for *Essence of Care*.

Activity 6.8 Factors to consider

What factors would you consider before and after a patient has used the toilet, or have been in contact with bodily fluids?
Always think about standard precautions, such as washing your hands before and after assisting your patient to use the toilet. Always use gloves and apron if you are likely to come into contact with bodily fluids, and remember to offer hand-washing facilities for your patient. Gloves should be worn for invasive procedures, any contact with sterile sites, non-intact skin, mucous membranes and exposure to blood, body fluids and sharp or contaminated instruments (Flores, 2007).

Activity 6.9 Communication skills

What communication skills would you use when caring for a patient with elimination needs?

- Observation
- Listening
- Approachability

(continued)

Activity 6.9 (Continued)

- Good non-verbal communication skills
- Being able to recognise non-verbal cues
- Professionalism
- Non jargon and appropriate use of language

Activity 6.10 Barriers to communication

What barriers to communication could cause elimination problems?

- Embarrassment
- Humiliation
- Physical illness
- Patients with
  - mental health or learning disabilities
  - communication difficulties (see Activity 6.2)

Activity 6.11 Common words used

Poo, passing stool, number 2 and many more!!! Be aware of cultural differences in terminology as well.

Activity 6.12 Diagram

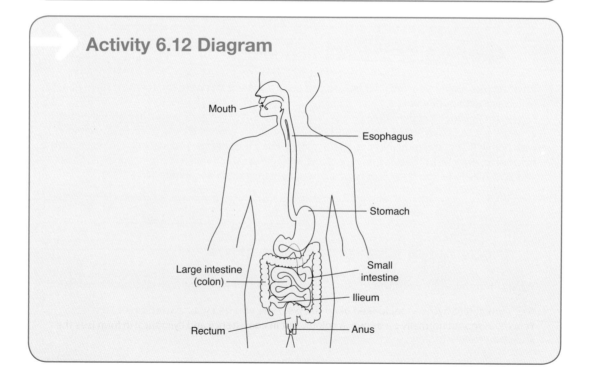

Mouth

Esophagus

Stomach

Large intestine (colon)

Small intestine

Ilieum

Rectum

Anus

Activity 6.13 Key words

Key word	Function
Mouth	The mouth is the start of the alimentary canal or GI tract. It receives food and the mechanical breakdown of food particle begins here.
Oesophagus	The oesophagus is a muscular tube approx. 25 cm long running from the pharynx to the stomach.
Stomach	This is a J-shaped muscular organ situated below the diaphragm. The stomach expands and stores food and normally empties its contents in 2–6 h.
Large intestine	The large intestine is also known as the colon. It is divided into the ascending, transverse, descending and sigmoid colons. Its function is the absorption of water, secrete mucin, prepare cellulose and defaecation. Its length is 1.5 m (Marieb, 2004) which is shorter than the small intestine.
Small intestine	The small intestine is much smaller that the large intestine and extends from the pyloric sphincter to the ileocaecal valve of the large intestine and is about 6 m in length.
Rectum	The rectum in the adult is usually 10–15 cm in length with the distal end called the anus (Kozier *et al.*, 2004). The rectum stores solid waste until it leaves the body through the anus. The word rectum comes from the Latin 'rectus' meaning straight (which the human rectum is not).
The anal canal	The anal canal is bounded by an external sphincter muscle which is voluntarily controlled and internal sphincter muscle which is involuntarily controlled (Kozier *et al.*, 2004).

Source: Adapted from Nair (2005).

Activity 6.14 What your stool should look like?

Write down what your stool looked liked the last time you had your bowels open.
Your stool should normally be brown in colour, soft in consistency and cylindrical in form (see the Bristol Stool Chart). The smell should not be offensive.

Activity 6.15 Foods affecting your stool

What foods affect your stool and why?
The food you eat and drink provides your body with many nutrients. These nutrients give you energy and help you stay healthy. As food moves through your body, it breaks down so that the nutrients can enter your body. This process is called digestion. After the food is digested, the leftover waste products move into the large intestine. Here water is removed, leaving stool or faecal matter. The stool moves into the last part of the large intestine, called the colon or bowel. As the bowel fills with stool it stretches. This triggers messages to the body. One message starts muscles to move the stool down through the bowel. Another message lets you know it is time to go to the bathroom and controls the muscle at the opening of the rectum (anus). This muscle allows you to control when the waste (stool) leaves the body. This is then called a bowel movement. The type of food that is in your diet has a very big effect on your body and especially on your stool. The amount of fibre in your diet will affect the amount, texture and how often you need to go to the toilet. Fibre is the fibrous or stringy part of fruit, vegetables and cereals that soaks up water in your intestines and produces a soft easy to pass stool as it is not digested. Some foods can pass through your body without being broken down in such a way that they can be seen in your stool. Sweet corn, tomato pips and skins, poppy seeds can all be seen. Some foods can colour your stool, such as beetroot and curry.

Activity 6.16 Constituents of stool

Write here what you think your stool consists of.
Normal faeces are made up of 75% water and 25% solid constituents. This is made up from cellulose, dead epithelial tissue, bacteria, mucous and bile pigments. They are normally semisolid in consistency and also contain inorganic matter (Tortora and Grabowski, 2002). Skatole and Indole arise from bacterial composition which gives faeces its characteristic smell. The average adult passes around 100–150 gm/day, though this varies from person to person.

Activity 6.17 Factors to consider

Write down what you should consider when observing your patient's stool.

- Amount
- Frequency
- Consistency
- Colour
- Pain
- Flatus (wind) (Nicol and Bavin, 2003).

Activity 6.18 Predisposing factors causing constipation

Write down the possible causes why a patient could suffer from constipation.

- Poor dietary habits
- Highly refined diet with little fibre
- Poor fluid intake
- Lack of exercise
- Neurological disorders, such as multiple sclerosis
- Diseases of the large bowel, e.g. tumours, adhesions, diverticular disease and anal strictures.
- Opioid drugs such as morphine (LeMone and Burke, 2004)
- Psychological symptoms, e.g. depression
- Clinical signs and symptoms such as:
  - Abdominal pain
  - Abdominal distension
  - Loss of appetite
  - Nausea and vomiting
  - Hard and dry faecal matter (if produced). (Nair, 2005)

Activity 6.19 Prevention of constipation

What factors would you consider when giving information to a patient in the prevention of constipation?
Factors to consider could be:

- Financial: Is there enough money for healthy foods?
- Oral: Are there any problems with your patient's teeth or dentures that may affect healthy eating? Do they have any infections in their mouth?
- Are they drinking enough water?
- Do they have enough fibre in their diet?
- Are they taking any medication that may cause constipation? For example, some analgesics, morphine, antidiarrhoeal medication or antacids.
- Are they doing enough exercise?
- What are their bowel habits and do they ignore the urge to pass stool?

Activity 6.20 Position of patient

What position would you place a patient before administering a suppository and why?
The patient must be positioned on the left (lateral) side with the knees flexed; the upper leg higher than the lower leg, and the buttocks close to the edge of the bed. This allows ease of passage of the suppository into the rectum by following the natural anatomy of the colon. Flexing the knees will reduce the discomfort as the suppository is passed through the anal sphincter. Ensure that you read your local policy of the procedure for the administration of a suppository.

Activity 6.21 Advice to patient

What advice would you give to your patient after administering a suppository?
You would inform your patient that this glycerol suppository may give them abdominal pain and to try to hold on to the suppository for at least 15–20 min. You should leave the commode and call bell nearby.

Activity 6.22 Observation of stool

Write down what you would observe for when a patient experiences a bout of acute diarrhoea.
Any blood or excess mucous in the stool should be reported and documented. Mucous is naturally produced to protect the bowel and will be present in faeces. Excess mucous may indicate bowel disease and should be investigated. Pale, clay consistency stool (steatorrhoea) may suggest biliary tract disease. Black, tarry, offensive smelling stool (melaena) indicates high bleeding in the gastro-intestinal tract. Fresh blood suggests disease or local pathology of the lower intestinal tract. Passive soiling may be due to weak anal sphincters or low puborectalis muscle tone. Any pain or discomfort when passing stools can be due to a variety of causes, which may be identified on physical examination, such as haemorrhoids or anal fissure.

Activity 6.23 Causes of diarrhoea

List some disorders that could cause chronic diarrhoea.
Most diarrhoea is caused by colonic disease, and in the absence of clinical evidence for malabsorption, initial investigations should focus on the lower gastro-intestinal tract (Metcalf, 2007). However, diarrhoea can also be caused by bacterial and viral infections and food poisoning. Bacteria or viruses may have been transmitted from person to person; so for this reason, it is important to wash your hands with soap and water after using the toilet and offer the same for your patient. Diarrhoea occurs when the microorganisms irritate the mucous membrane of the small or large intestine resulting in an abnormally large quantity of water in the motions. The irritated gut becomes very active, contracting excessively and irregularly (colic). This can be accompanied by nausea, vomiting and cold sweats. In some cases, the motions may include some blood. Certain bacteria (usually staphylococci) irritate the digestive tract by producing toxins. These toxins affect the mucous membrane much sooner, a few hours after consumption, compared with bacterial infection. When taking antibiotics, many people suffer from diarrhoea, which may continue after the antibiotic course has finished. The diarrhoea occurs because the antibiotic alters the intestinal bacterial environment, so cannot be classed as an allergic reaction. Twenty percent of cases suffer from diarrhoea as a result of broad spectrum antibiotic therapy such as Ampicillin; however, the incidence is lower when taking Amoxicillin, which is better absorbed (Spiller, 1994).
Chronic diarrhoea can be a symptom of many disorders such as:

● Irritable bowel syndrome
● Inflammatory bowel diseases such as ulcerative colitis, Crohn's disease or coeliac disease
● Chronic pancreatitis
● Laxatives

Activity 6.23 (Continued)

- Diet — lactose/gluten intolerance
- Metabolic disorders such as diabetes or thyrotoxicosis
- Drugs and alcohol (adapted from Thomas *et al.*, 2003; Metcalf, 2007)

Activity 6.24 Nursing care

What nursing care would be required for a patient suffering from chronic diarrhoea?

- Skin care, particularly around the anal area (read Norton and Kamm, 1999)
- Physical assessment
- Nutrition and fluid replacement (read Metcalf, 2007)
- Psychological and emotional support

Activity 6.25

List here the functions of the kidney.

- To excrete urine and waste products such as urea, uric acid and creatinine
- To regulate electrolyte balance
- To maintain pH of the blood
- To secrete rennin, which helps to regulate blood pressure
- To secrete erythropoietin, which stimulates the production of red blood cells (Nair, 2005)

Activity 6.26 The urinary system

Label the diagram of the urinary tract. The key words are here to help you to complete the diagram.

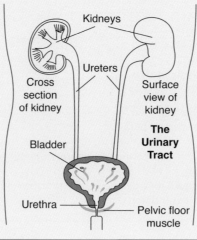

Kidneys

Ureters

Cross section of kidney

Surface view of kidney

The Urinary Tract

Bladder

Urethra

Pelvic floor muscle

Activity 6.27 Key terms

Now identify the meaning of each of these words.

Key term	Definition
Haematuria	Blood in the urine
Glycosuria	Glucose in the urine
Micturition	It is also known as urinating or voiding
Ketonuria	Ketones in the urine
Proteinuria	Protein in the urine
Anuria	Lack of urine production
Dysuria	Voiding that is painful or difficult
Oliguria	Low urine output
Polyuria or diuresis	Production of large amounts of urine
Acute urinary retention	The sudden inability to pass urine and is often associated with severe abdominal pain (Thomas et al., 2005).

Activity 6.28

What else do you think can cause UTI?
Another cause of bladder infections or UTI can be waiting too long to urinate. The bladder is a muscle that stretches to hold urine and contracts when the urine is released. Waiting very long past the time you first feel the need to urinate causes the bladder to stretch beyond its capacity, which over time can weaken the bladder muscle. When the bladder is weakened, it may not empty completely and some urine is left in the bladder which may increase the risk of UTI or bladder infection.

Activity 6.29 Factors predisposing to UTI

What factors predispose patients to UTIs?
Factors that predispose or cause UTI could be:

- Women are more susceptible that men
- Urethral contamination from bowel flora
- Previous history of UTI
- Sexual activity, especially with new partner or vigorous intercourse
- Delayed postcoital urination
- Anatomical or structural factors, for example uterine prolapse or oestrogen deficiency
- Instrumentation such as catheterisation (Anderson, 1999).

Activity 6.30 The role of the nurse

Describe the role of the nurse in the management of a UTI.

- Assessment
- Measurement and documentation
- Maintain privacy and dignity
- Maintain universal precautions
- Promote fluid intake
- Maintain normal toileting habits
- Assist with toileting if required
- Prevention of future UTI
- Promote continence through education

Activity 6.31 Urinalysis and its purpose

Describe in your own words what urinalysis is and the purpose of this assessment?
Urinalysis is a non-invasive collection of urine and is the physical and/or chemical examination of urine. It consists of a range of chemical and microscopic tests to screen for UTIs, renal disease and diseases of other organs that result in the appearance of abnormal metabolites (breakdown products) in the urine. Urine testing can supply you with knowledge that will provide you with information about the health of your patient and you will be able to test for substances that are not usually found in urine such as blood and glucose. However, urinalysis should not be used in isolation to guide treatment, for example if urine is left to stand or is contaminated, a false reading could occur, thereby increasing the risk of for inaccurate results. Read Wilson (2005) for further discussion on urinalysis and using reagent strips.

Activity 6.32 Component of urine

What do you think the main component of urine is and what should a normal specimen look like?

- 96% water
- 2% urea
- 2% uric acid, creatinine, sodium, potassium, chlorides, phosphates, sulfates and oxalates
- Colour ranges from yellow to amber but depends on the concentration, some drugs or food dyes.
- There should not be a strong odour and should be clear when voided (Pollard and Levy, 2005).
- Haematuria is the term to describe blood in the urine and could be suggestive of disease or damage to the renal system (Selfe, 2006).

Activity 6.33 Factors that affect urine output

What factors may increase or decrease urine output?

- *Fluid intake*. The amount of fluid that a person takes in has a direct correlation with the amount of fluid the body excretes
- *Medications*. Diuretics may lead to an increase of urinary output
- *Caffeine and sodium*. Foods and fluids containing caffeine may increase urinary output, whilst food containing high amounts of sodium may cause a decrease in urinary output.
- *Urinary diversions*. Patients who have urinary diversions such as indwelling catheters may have urine that is normally cloudy, with large amounts of sediments (Evans-Smith, 2005).

Activity 6.34 Glycosuria

What is the commonest cause of glucose found in a patient's urine?
Glycosuria refers to the presence of glucose in the urine. Glucose should not normally be detected in urine. Glucose in the urine indicates high blood glucose levels and may be indicative of undiagnosed or uncontrolled diabetes mellitus (Kozier *et al.*, 2008).

Activity 6.35 Reflection

Reflect on your placement experiences when dealing with elimination needs of a patient. Write in sentences what happened, how did it make you feel and what would you do differently (if anything) next time when the patient requires assistance with elimination.

What happened?

- Describe the scenario briefly relating to your learning need.

How did it make you feel?

- Did you feel good or bad about it?
- What was good or bad about the situation?
- Did you have adequate underpinning knowledge to carry out the care?
- If you had previous experience of similar situation, was it useful this time?

What would you do differently (if anything) next time?

- Has this personal experience encouraged you to do further reading

This is only a guide. Please address the sub-headings to meet your own learning needs.

References

Abd-El-Maeboud, K., El-Naggar, T., El-Hawi, E., Mahmoud, S. and Abd-El-Hay, S. (1991) Rectal suppository: commonsense and mode of insertion. *The Lancet* **338**, 798–800.

Anderson, R.U. (1999) Management of lower urinary tract infections and cystitis. *The Urologic Clinics of North America* **26** (4), 729–735.

Ayliffe, G.A.J., Babb, J.R. and Taylor, L.J. (1999) *Hospital-Acquired Infection. Principles and Prevention*, 3rd edn (Oxford: Butterworth-Heinemann).

Baillie, L. (ed.) (2001) *Developing Practical Nursing Skills* (London: Arnold).

Baillie, L. and Arrowsmith, V. (2005) Meeting elimination needs. In *Developing Practical Nursing Skills*, L. Baillie, ed. (London: Hodder Arnold).

Barrett, J. (2002) Pathophysiology of constipation and faecal incontinence in older people. In *Bowel Care in Older People*, J. Potter, C. Norton and A. Cottenden, eds (Sudbury: Royal College of Physicians).

Bashe, A. (1987) Symptom distress changes in elimination. *Semin Oncol Nurs* **3** (4), 287–292.

Bisanz, A. (2007) Chronic constipation. *American Journal of Nursing* **107** (4), 72 B–72 H.

Bradshaw, A. and Price, L. (2007) Rectal suppository insertion: the reliability of the evidence as a basis for nursing practice. *Journal of Clinical Nursing* **16** (1), 98–103.

Cadd, A., Keatinge, D. and Henssen, M. (2000) Assessment and documentation of bowel care management in palliative care: incorporating patient preferences into the care regimen. *Journal of Clinical Nursing* **9**, 228–235.

Carr, B. (1996) Assessing incontinence. *Practice Nursing* **7** (2), 19–23.

Chiasson, J.L, Aris-Jilwan, N. and Belanger, R. (2003) Diagnosis and treatment of diabetic ketoacidocis and hyperglycaemic hyperosmolar state. *Canadian Medical Association Journal* **168** (7), 859–866.

Department of Health (2000) *The NHS Plan*, DH (London: The Stationery Office).

Department of Health (2001) *The Essence of Care: Patient-Focused Benchmarks for Clinical Governance* (London: The Stationery Office).

Dougherty, L. and Lister, S. (2008) *The Royal Marsden Manual of Clinical Nursing Procedures*, 7th edn (Oxford: Blackwell).

Edwards, C. (1997) Down and away: an overview of adult constipation and faecal incontinence. In *Promoting Continence: A Clinical and Research Resource*, K. Getliffe and M. Dolman, eds (London: Balliere Tindall), pp. 77–226.

Edwards, S. (2001) Regulation of water, sodium and potassium: implications for practice. *Nursing Standard* **15** (22), 36–45.

Evans-Smith, P. (2005) *Taylor's Clinical Nursing Skills: A Nursing Process Approach* (Philadelphia: Lippincott Williams & Wilkins).

Flanning, H. (2000) Fluid and electrolyte balance. In *Surgical Nursing: Advancing Practice*, K. Manley and L. Bellman, eds (Edinburgh: Churchill Livingstone).

Flores, A. (2007) Appropriate glove use in the prevention of cross-infection. *Nursing Standard* **21** (35), 45–48.

Gill, D. (1999) Practical procedures for nurses. stool specimen. 1. assessment. *Nursing Times* **95**, 26.

Health Protection Agency (2005) Investigation of urine: National standard method. BSOP. 41, 5. www.hpa-standardmethods.org.uk (accessed 22 February 2008).

Henke, K. and Eigsti, J. (2003) Renal physiology: review and practical application in the critically ill patient. *Dimensions of Critical Care Nursing* **22** (3), 125–132.

Hill, S. (2006) Microbiology and antibiotic resistance of urinary tract infections. *Trends in Urology, Gynaecology and Sexual Health* **11**(3), 26–31.

Hilton, P.A. (ed.) (2004) *Fundamental Nursing Skills* (London: Whurr).

Hogan, C.M. (1998) The nurses' role in diarrhoea management. *Oncol Nurses Forum* **25** (5), 879–886.

Human Rights Act (1998) http://www.direct.gov.uk/en/RightsAndResponsibilities/Citizensandgovernment/DG_4002951 (accessed 1 February 2008).

Kauffman, T.L. (1999) *Geriatric Rehabilitation Manual* (New York: Churchill Livingstone).

Koch, T & Kelly, S (1999) Identifying strategies for managing urinary incontinence with women who have multiple sclerosis. *Journal of Clinical Nursing* **8** (5), 550–559.

Kozier, B., Erb, G., Berman, A. and Synder, S.J. (2004) *Fundamentals of Nursing*, 7th edn (Englewood Cliffs: Pearson Prentice Hall).

Kozier, B., Erb, G., Berman, A., Snyder, S., Lake, R. and Harvey, S. (2008) *Fundamentals of Nursing: Concepts, Process and Practice* (Pearson Education).

Kyle, G. (2006) Assessment and treatment of older people with constipation. *Nursing Standard* **21** (8), 41–46.

LeMone, P. and Burke, K.M. (2004) *Medical Surgical Nursing: Critical Thinking in Client Care*, 3rd edn (Upper Saddle River: Prentice Hall).

Mader, S.S. (1997) *Understanding Human Anatomy and Physiology*, 3rd edn (London: Wm C. Brown).

Marieb, E.N. (2004) *Human Anatomy and Physiology*, 6th edn (London: Addison Wesley).

McGhee, M. (2004) Lab investigations. *Practice Nurse* **28** (9), 19–26.

Metcalf, C. (2007) Chronic diarrhoea: investigation, treatment and nursing care. *Nursing Standard* **21** (21), 48–56.

Nair, M. (2005) Elimination: alimentary and urinary tracts. In *Compendium of Clinical Skills for Student Nurses*, I. Peate, ed. (London: Whurr).

Naish, W. and Hallam, M. (2007) Urinary tract infection: diagnosis and management for nurses. *Nursing Standard* **21** (23), 50–57.

Neno, R. and Neno, M. (2006) Promoting a healthy diet for older people in the community. *Nursing Standard* **20** (29), 59–65.

Nicol, M. and Bavin, C. (2003) *Essential Nursing Skills* (Elsevier Health Sciences).

Norton, C. (2006) Perianal skin care. *Gastrointestinal Nursing* **4** (1), 18–25.

Norton, C. and Kamm, M. (1999) *Bowel Control: Information and Practical Advice* (Beaconsfield: Beaconsfield Publishers).

Nursing and Midwifery Council (2004) *Standards of Proficiency for Pre-Registration Nursing Education* (London: Nursing and Midwifery Council).

Nursing and Midwifery Council (2005) *Guidelines for Records and Record Keeping* (London: Nursing and Midwifery Council).

Nursing and Midwifery Council (2007) *The Essential Skills Clusters*, Annexe 1, (London: Nursing and Midwifery Council).

Nursing and Midwifery Council (2008) *The Code: Standards of Conduct, Performance and Ethics for Nurses and Midwives* (London: Nursing and Midwifery Council).

Pollard, C. and Levy, B. (2005) *Eliminating*. In *Fundamental Nursing Skills*, P.E. Hilton, ed. (London, Philadelphia: Whurr).

Prodigy Guidance (2008) *Constipation*. http://www.cks.library.nhs.uk/constipation/view_whole_topic_review (accessed 15 March 2008).

Richmond, J. (2003) Prevention of constipation through risk management. *Nursing Standard* **17** (16), 39–46.

Roper, N., Logan, W. and Tierney, A. (1990) *The Elements of Nursing: A Model of Living*, 3rd edn (Edinburgh: Churchill Livingstone).

Rowell, D.M. (1998) Evaluation of urine chemistry analyser. *Professional Nurse* **13**, 553–554.

Royal College of Nursing (2008) http://rcnlz.axiainteractive.net/default.aspx (accessed 26 June 2008). (You will need your RCN membership number and password for this site.)

Royal Pharmaceutical Society of Great Britain and British Medical Association (2008) *British National Formulary 56* (London: Pharmaceutical Press).

Sander, R. (2007) Urinary tract infections. *Nursing Older People* **19** (3), 38–39.

Selfe, L. (2006) The urinary system. In *Nursing Practice – Hospital and Home: The Adult*, 3rd edn, M. Alexander, J. Fawcett and P. Runciman, eds (Edinburgh: Churchill Livingstone).

Sinclair, A. and Woodhouse, K. (1995) *Acute Medical Illness in Old Age* (London: Chapman and Hall Medical).

Smith, S.F. (2001) Evidence-based management of constipation in the oncology patient. *European Journal of Oncology Nursing* **5** (1), 18–25.

Smith, S.F., Duell, D.J. and Martin, B.C. (2004) *Clinical Nursing Skills: Basic to Advanced Skills*, 6th edn (New Jersey: Prentice Hall).

Spiller, R. (1994) *Diarrhoea and Constipation* (London: Science Press).

Steggall, M.J. (2007a) Urine samples and urinalysis. *Nursing Standard* **22** (14–16), 42–45.

Steggall, M.J. (2007b) Acute urinary retention: causes, clinical features and patient care. *Nursing Standard* **21** (29), 42–46.

Tarling, C. (1997) Toileting and clothing. In *The Guide to Handling of Patients: Introducing a Safer Handling Policy*, 4th edn (London: National Back Pain Association), pp. 163–171.

Tenorio, A.R., Badri, S.M. and Sahgal, N.B. (2001) Effectiveness of gloves in the prevention of hand carriage of vancomycin-resistant enterococcus species by health care workers after patient care. *Clinical Infectious Diseases* **32** (5), 826–829.

Thomas, K., Oades, G., Taylor-Hay, C. and Kirby, R.S. (2005) Acute urinary retention: what is the impact on patients' quality of life? *British Journal of Urology International* **95** (1), 72–76.

Thomas, P.D., Forbes, A. and Green, J. (2003) Guidelines for the investigation for chronic diarrhoea. *Gut* **52** (Suppl. 5), V1–15.

Tortora, G.A. and Grabowski, S.R. (2002) *Principles of Anatomy and Physiology* (New York: John Wiley and Sons).

Walsh, K. and Kowanko, I. (2002) Nurses' and patients' perceptions of dignity. *International Journal of Nursing Practice* **8** (3), 143–151.

Wilson, L.A. (2005) Urinalysis. *Nursing Standard* **19** (35), 51–54.

Woogara, J. (2004) *An Ethnographic Study of Privacy of the Person in National Health Service Patient Care Settings, with Reference to Human Rights.* Unpublished thesis, Guildford, University of Surrey.

Further reading

Baillie, L. (2000) *Developing Practice Nursing Skills* (London: Arnold).

Bradshaw, A. and Price, L. (2007) Rectal suppository insertion: the reliability of the evidence as a basis for nursing practice. *Journal of Clinical Nursing* **16**, 98–103.

Boyd-Carson, W. (2003) Faecal incontinence in adults. *Nursing Standard* **18** (8), 42–55, 54.

Christer, R. *et al.* (2003) Constipation: causes and cures. *Nursing Times* **99** (25), 26–27.

Chung, L. *et al.* (2002) The efficiency of fluid balance charting: an evidence-based management project. *Journal of Nursing Management* **10** (2), 103–113.

Cook, R. (1996) Urinalysis: ensuring accurate urine testing. *Nursing Standard* **10** (46), 49–52.

Dosh, S. (2002) Evaluation and treatment of constipation. *The Journal of Family Practice* **51** (6), 555–560.

Dougherty, L. and Lister, S. (2008) *The Royal Marsden Manual of Clinical Nursing Procedures*, 7th edn (Oxford: Blackwell).

Grey, M., Ratcliffe, C. and Donovan, A. (2002) Perineal skin care for the incontinent patient. *Advance in Skin Wound Care* **4**, 170–175.

Hilton, P.A. (2004) *Fundamental Nursing Skills* (London: Whurr).

Metcalf, M. (2007) Chronic diarrhoea: investigation, treatment and nursing care. *Nursing Standard* **21** (21), 48–56.

Moppet, S. (2000) Which way is up for a suppository? *Nursing Times Plus* **96** (19), 12–13.

Peate, I. (2003) Nursing role in the management of constipation: use of laxatives. *British Journal of Nursing* **12**, 1130–1136.

Richmond, J. (2003) Prevention of constipation through risk management. *Nursing Standard* **17**(16), 39–46.

Rigby, D. (2000) Management of bowel dysfunction: evacuation difficulties. *Nursing Standard* **14** (47), 47–51.

Rigby, D. (2005) Understanding urine testing. *Nursing Times* **101** (12), 60–62.

Stiwell, B. (1993) Assessing the adult with constipation. *Skills Update-Book 2* (London: Macmillan).

Ward, D. (2003) Improving patient hand hygiene. *Nursing Standard* **17** (35) 39–42.

Wells, M. (1997) Urinalysis. *Professional Nurse Study Supplement* Nov 13(2), 11–13.

7 Principles of skin care

JULIE VUOLO

→ Aims

The aim of this chapter is to introduce the key principles of good skin care and provide an overview of the care of patients who have common skin-related problems.

→ Learning objectives

On completion of this chapter, you will learn to:
- Describe the anatomical structure of the skin
- Identify the core functions of the skin
- Know how to care for the skin
- Understand why good skin care is one of the key elements of essential nursing care
- Demonstrate an awareness of common skin-related problems
- Understand how the key themes of communication, privacy and dignity and health and safety, relate to the principles of good skin care

---

Introduction

Caring for the skin is an essential skill for any healthcare worker. It is the largest organ of the body comprising 16% of the total body weight (Knight, 2003) and it performs multiple functions in the body. Skin health is affected by internal factors such as disease, dehydration and poor nutrition. It is also vulnerable to damage from external factors such as physical trauma, harmful microorganisms and adverse environmental conditions.

To care for the skin properly, you need to first understand its anatomy (structure) and function. This will help you to understand the role the skin plays in the body and what effect damaging the skin has. Understanding the structure and function of the skin is the first step to providing good skin care.

Activity 7.1 Key terms

Use your nursing dictionary to complete the glossary below; this is good preparation for reading the rest of the chapter.

Term	Definition
Abrasion	
Arrector pili	
Callus	
Capillary	
Carotene	
Chloracne	
Connective tissue	
Epidermis	
Dermis	
Diabetic neuropathy	
Haemoglobin	
Hypodermis	
Irritant contact dermatitis	
Keratinocytes	
Laceration	
Lipid	
Melanin	

→ Activity 7.1 (*Continued*)

Microorganism	
Oedema	
Pigment	
Puncture wound	
Sebaceous glands	
Sebum	
Shearing force	
Stratum basale	
Stratum corneum	
Stratum granulosum	
Stratum lucidum	
Stratum spinosum	
Sudoriferous glands	
Tensile strength	
Turgor	
Vasoconstriction	
Vasodilation	

Anatomy of the skin

The skin is comprised of two layers, the epidermis (top layer) and dermis (deeper layer). These two layers are anchored by the hypodermis. In adults, the skin covers an area of about 2 m^2 and weighs between 4.5 and 5 kg (Jenkins *et al.*, 2007). The skin is about 1–2 mm thick, although this varies according to the site, from 0.5 mm on the eyelids to 4.0 mm on the heels (Jenkins *et al.*, 2007).

The epidermis

The epidermis is made up of a number of different layers. Can you name them all?

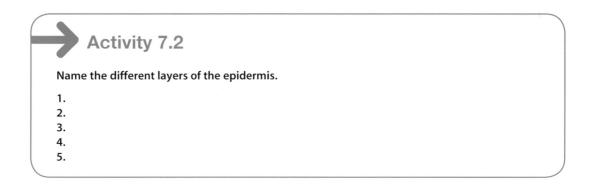

Activity 7.2

Name the different layers of the epidermis.

1.
2.
3.
4.
5.

The deepest layer of the epidermis is the stratum basale from which new epidermal skin cells (keratinocytes) arise. New cells move upwards through the layers of the epidermis changing as they do so. As they reach near the surface of the skin, they become less active and eventually die. The stratum corneum, or outer layer, is simply an accumulation of dead keratinocyte cells, about 25–30 layers in total. These cells are continually shed (ever wondered where house dust comes from?) to be replaced by more layers of cells pushing their way up from deeper down. The life cycle of a keratinocyte cell from its 'birth' in the stratum basale to its eventually death in the stratum corneum is on average about 4 weeks (Jenkins *et al.*, 2007).

Although the stratum corneum is comprised of dead cells, it still serves an important function in protecting the deeper, active skin cells from damage. In addition, the stratum corneum has a high lipid content which acts as an effective waterproof barrier.

The dermis

The dermis is made mainly of connective tissue and contains blood vessels, nerves, sensory receptors, hair follicles and lymphatic vessels and glands. It is divided into two regions: the papillary region and reticular region.

The papillary region of the dermis lies beneath the epidermis and contains capillary loops (small blood vessels) and receptors which are sensitive to touch and nerve endings which initiate signals which produce sensations such as warmth, pain and itching. The reticular region of the dermis lies beneath the papillary region and is attached to the hypodermis. It contains small blood vessels, nerves, hair follicles, sudoriferous and sebaceous glands. The strength and elasticity of the type of tissue in the reticular region give the skin its ability to stretch, as well as return to shape afterwards.

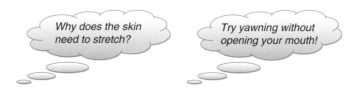

Skin colour

Skin colour is determined by three pigments: carotene, haemoglobin and melanin. Haemoglobin, the oxygen carrying pigment found in the blood, gives a pinkish/red tint to the skin, and carotene, which is a precursor of vitamin A, gives a yellow/orange tone. Melanin, found mainly in the epidermis, causes the skin to vary from very pale to very dark in colour. Melanin is produced by cells called melanocytes and it is the amount of melanin produced by the melanocytes rather than the number of melanocytes that determines the colour of the skin. Freckles and age spots (sometimes called liver spots) are just dense patches of melanin. Safe exposure to sunlight stimulates melanin production giving the skin a tanned appearance and providing some protection from ultraviolet (UV) radiation.

Types of skin

There are variations in the exact structure and function of the skin depending on site. Because of these variations, two main types of skin are recognized: thin skin (hairy) and thick skin (hairless). Try Activity 7.3 before you read on.

> ## ➜ Activity 7.3
>
> **Where on the body do you think you might find *thin* skin?**
>
>
> **Where on the body do you think you might find *thick* skin?**

Now read on to find out if you were right! *Thin* (hairy) skin covers all parts of the body except the palms (including the palmar surface of the fingers) and the soles of the feet. Thin skin has hair and sebaceous (oil) glands but fewer sudoriferous (sweat) glands. Thin skin also has fewer sensory receptors than thick skin. Overall, the epidermis of thin skin is between 0.10 and 0.15 mm (Jenkins *et al.*, 2007).

The palms of the hands, palmar surface of the fingers and the soles of the feet are covered by *thick* (hairless) skin. Thick skin therefore has no hair or arrector pili muscles (more about these later), nor does it have sebaceous glands. However, thick skin has more sudoriferous glands and more sensory receptors than thin skin. The epidermis of thick skin is between 0.6 and 4.5 mm (Jenkins *et al.*, 2007). Thick skin is also characterised by the presence of epidermal ridges, a series of ridges and grooves appearing as lines, loops or whorls on the outer layer. These ridges are downward projections of the epidermis into the dermis. They increase the surface area of the skin and therefore the ability of the skin to grip by means of friction.

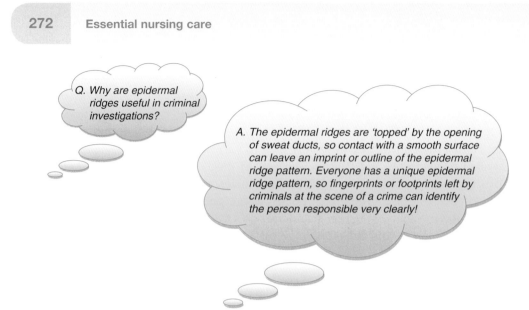

Now, before reading further, try Activity 7.4.

Activity 7.4

Can you accurately label this diagram of the skin?

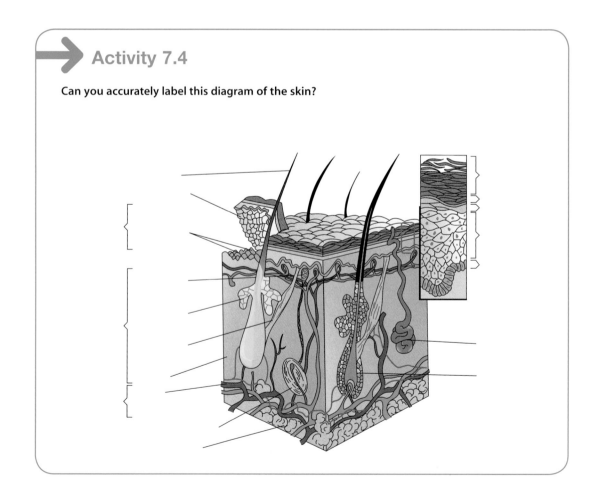

Functions of the skin

The skin has numerous functions which are all important in maintaining body health. In this section, we will look at the key functions of the skin.

Protection

The intact skin acts as a physical barrier to protect internal organs and tissues from damage by a variety of harmful external factors such as UV light, toxins and mechanical damage. As an external organ, the skin is subjected to many traumatic episodes throughout a lifetime but this is nothing compared to the damage to internal organs if they were exposed instead. For this reason, the skin has considerable tensile strength and a high resilience to accidental damage. Tensile strength is the ability of any material (including the skin) to tolerate a force which pulls it in two opposite directions. For example, tissue paper (low tensile) tears easily when pulled in opposite directions but nylon thread (high tensile) does not. Try it for yourself at home using different materials. The skin must be able to resist this kind of force or pressure because it is subjected to it regularly.

Activity 7.5

Think about tensile strength. List three examples of when skin might be subjected to a pulling force.

1.
2.
3.

The skin is also very resilient to direct damage. If we knock ourselves, we may bruise but the skin will usually stay intact (i.e. in one piece) and in place. Imagine if every time you accidentally knocked yourself, a piece of your skin fell off!

Maintenance of body temperature

The human body functions best at 37°C (Watson, 2000); if it becomes either too hot or too cold, essential activity such as brain or heart function is affected. The skin plays a key role in maintaining the ideal body temperature by warming and cooling the body as required and it does this in two ways. To cool the body, the blood vessels supplying the skin are made larger (vasodilation) resulting in an increase in blood flow to the skin tissues. As the warm blood reaches the surface of the skin, it is cooled by six different mechanisms (Watson, 2000); these mechanisms are radiation, conduction, convection, evaporation, respiration and excretion.

→ **Activity 7.6**

Find out the definitions of each of the six blood cooling mechanisms.

Mechanism	Definition
Radiation	
Conduction	
Convection	
Evaporation	
Respiration	
Excretion	

Conversely, to warm the body the same blood vessels are made smaller (vasoconstriction). As the amount of blood flowing to the skin is reduced, the heat is retained internally instead. Secondly, much of the skin is covered in fine hairs. When the body requires cooling, these hairs lay flat in order to prevent the trapping of any warmth being radiated from the skin surface; warm air can then evaporate swiftly. When the body requires warming, the hairs stand upright so that warm air radiating from the skin surface can be trapped in a layer around the body and evaporation is minimised; this is usually accompanied by lots of shivering which also produces heat to help warm you up — brrr!

The position of the hairs is controlled by a small muscle in the skin called the arrector pili muscle which relaxes to allow the hairs to fall flat and contracts to bring them upright.

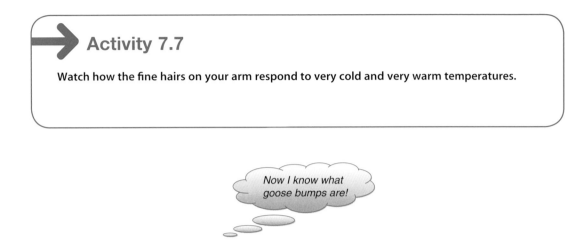

Activity 7.7

Watch how the fine hairs on your arm respond to very cold and very warm temperatures.

Now I know what goose bumps are!

Barrier to infection

The skin provides a physical barrier to infection by stopping potentially harmful microorganisms to gain internal access. When the skin barrier is broken, for example when cut, these microorganisms can wreak havoc internally by causing either infection or disease. A further barrier to microorganism damage is provided by the presence of sweat and sebum on the skin surface. The components of these have a pH of between 4.5 and 6 (Hughes, 2001), which makes the skin slightly acidic. The acidic environment of the skin may play a role in defending the body against pathogenic microorganisms which would flourish under more alkaline conditions. This protective function of the acid barrier led to the use of the term 'acid mantle' as far back as the 1930s (Schmid and Korting, 1995).

Sensation

The skin is full of nerve endings. These nerve endings respond to external stimuli such as pain, temperature, texture and moisture. In healthy people, messages sent from these nerve endings to the brain are interpreted and acted upon quickly. This speed of this mechanism can protect us from harm or injury, for example, by withdrawing our hand from a surface because we can sense it is burning hot. External stimuli help us to interpret the world around us as well as protect us from harm.

Vitamin D production

The skin utilises sunlight to produce vitamin D (it is sometimes called the sunshine vitamin). This vitamin is essential for the development of healthy bones and teeth (Hughes, 2001). It cannot be manufactured without sunlight, a fact worth remember when caring for anybody who has been confined to indoors for many weeks.

Melanin production

The skin also produces the pigment melanin and protects it from harmful UV rays of the sunlight. However, prolonged exposure can result in skin cancers such as basal cell carninoma, squamous cell carninoma and malignant melanoma (Perfect *et al.*, 2001).

Communication

The skin plays an important role in self-image and communication with others. How we see ourselves and how others see us is often influenced by our outward physical appearance. The skin forms an essential part of how we look and whether we or others are happy with this will have significance in terms of our self-esteem. This can have both positive and negative effects on our ability to communicate effectively. But our skin is part of who we are, and unlike our kidneys or liver it is all on show for others to see!

Now try Activity 7.8

> ### ➡ Activity 7.8
>
> **Look at your face in the mirror. What words would you use to describe your skin?**

Healthy skin

Healthy skin is intact, well nourished and hydrated and disease free. Here are some of the commonest factors affecting skin health:

Age

As we grow older, our skin changes in many ways. It becomes less elastic as it loses some of its elastic fibres (Cua *et al.*, 1990). This can result in over-stretching of the skin tissues and damage from skin tearing and trauma. In addition, the epidermis becomes thinner (Baranoski and Ayello, 2004) and therefore more vulnerable to external types of mechanical injury such as friction. This type of skin injury is further exacerbated (worsened) by moisture. Moisture can arise from excess sweating, incontinence and insufficient drying of the skin.

The dermis also becomes thinner giving the skin a looser, more papery appearance (Jenkins *et al.*, 2007). As the dermis contains so many important structures, the loss of it affects these too. A reduction in blood vessels and nerve endings, for example, leads to poorer temperature control and decreased sensation. The number of sweat glands also reduces and the overall level of sebum produced decreases resulting in dryer skin. Dryness contributes to skin damage in a number of ways: by decreasing its ability to withstand stretching, by leading to cracks or fissures which can ulcerate (open into wounds) or become infected, by changing the skin pH to allow pathogenic (disease causing) bacteria to flourish.

In young skin, the epidermis and dermis are firmly adhered to each other but become less so as the skin ages. This weakness can result in separation of the two layers under force, particularly shearing type forces.

Environment

Both internal and external environments can be problematic for the skin. Indoors, central heating has a drying effect on the skin as do air conditioning units. People living or working for long periods in the very warm, dry atmospheres created by these systems may suffer from dry, itchy or flaky skin. Outdoors, weather conditions such as wind and cold may cause skin damage such as broken blood vessels, chapped lips and dry skin. Prolonged exposure to the sun (specifically UV radiation) can dry skin out and cause premature skin wrinkling and an increased risk of skin cancer (Perfect *et al.*, 2001). Environmental pollution can also have an impact resulting in skin problems such as chloracne and irritant contact dermatitis (English *et al.*, 2003).

Now look at Activity 7.9 and see if you can think of some examples of occupations which may expose the worker to damaging environments.

Activity 7.9

List three indoor (internal) occupations which may affect skin health.

1.
2.
3.

List three outdoor (external) occupations which may affect skin health.

1.
2.
3.

Nutrition (food) and hydration (drink)

The skin, like the rest of the body, needs foods from all the major food groups to function properly and regenerate new cells to replace dead or damaged ones. A healthy diet should include breads, potatoes and cereals and be rich in fruits and vegetables. It should also include moderate amounts of meat and fish (or meat/milk alternatives) and dairy products and limited amounts of foods containing fat or sugar (British Nutrition Foundation (BNF), 2003). Fluid is also essential for the body to work properly although the amount needed per day varies according to factors such as age, climate and activity (BNF, 2003).

Malnutrition occurs when an individual's nutrient intake falls below the requirements for normal cell function (National Prescribing Centre, 1998). Who do you think might be at risk of malnutrition? Try Activity 7.10.

Activity 7.10

Make a list of people who you think could be at risk of malnutrition.

1.   6.
2.   7.
3.   8.
4.   9.
5.   10.

Smoking

Smoking reduces the quality and quantity of blood flow to the skin (Waeber *et al.*, 1984; Tur *et al.*, 1992) leaving it more vulnerable to skin damage and delayed wound healing. It is also an important determinant in skin ageing and wrinkling (Leung and Harvey, 2002) so it doesn't do your looks any good either!

In this section, we have considered some of the factors affecting skin health. Now look at Activity 7.11 and think about how you could minimise the impact of some of these.

Activity 7.11

Air conditioning?	
Central heating?	
Smoking?	
Sun exposure?	
Poor nutrition?	
Poor hydration?	

In summary, the appearance of the skin tends to reflect the body's general state of health and the environment in which we live. Maximising skin health is one way to minimise the risk of skin damage, breakdown and disease. Remember, you cannot change the skin you have been given but you can look after it!

In the preceding sections, you have learned how the skin looks, what the skin does and what factors affect skin health. Now you are ready to move on to learn about skin assessment, skin hygiene and recognising and managing common skin problems.

Assessing the skin

It is important to assess the skin regularly for signs of skin damage or breakdown and for changes which may indicate the presence of disease. Remember, early detection of problems will maximise the chance to treat them successfully. Assessment of the skin should include finding out about the patient's normal skin condition and, with the patient's permission, carrying out a visual examination of the skin.

What questions to ask?

You need to ask questions that will encourage the patients to talk openly and confidently about themselves. Try a combination of open-ended and closed questions to ensure you get the information you need. Remember that closed questions lead the patients to respond with just a 'yes' or 'no'; if you were asking the patients whether they had ever had eczema, this would be the right kind of question to use. However, if you were asking them how they felt about having eczema, you would use an open-ended question to encourage a full and thoughtful answer. Here are some examples of questions you might ask:

'How would you describe your skin?' (open)
'Do you, or have you, ever suffered from a skin disorder or problem?' (closed)
'Does anybody in your family suffer from a skin disorder or problem?' (closed)
'How does having this skin disorder make you feel?' (open)
'Do you have any concerns or worries about your skin?' (closed)

When asking questions of this nature, remember to be sensitive to the feelings of your patient; this is particularly important if you are asking about disorders which are disfiguring or life threatening.

What to look for (visual examination)

When looking at the skin, consider the following headings: colour, texture, elasticity, temperature and integrity (continuity).

Colour

Skin colour varies according to the amount and type of pigment it contains (see Section 6). Skin colour alone is usually of little significance but changes in colour and patches of discolouration can be of importance. For example, a yellowing skin tone can indicate jaundice. Jaundice develops as a result of abnormally high blood levels of the bile pigment, bilirubin. Bilirubin is a by-product of breakdown of old red blood cells and it accumulates either when there are two many red blood cells being destroyed or when the mechanism for excreting it from the body is somehow damaged (Jenkins *et al.*, 2007). Jaundice can be an important indicator of underlying disease but it is worth noting that yellowing of the skin can also be caused by eating too many carrots!

Other skin colour changes include bluish/grey (can indicate insufficient oxygen in the blood stream), bright red skin (can indicate carbon monoxide poisoning) and pale/white (can indicate lack of sleep or sunlight or anaemia). Patches of discolouration may indicate a more localised problem such as an allergic rash, malignant (cancerous) mole or pressure damage. The temporary or permanent redness seen as a result of skin damage due to pressure, friction or shearing forces can be a pre-cursor to skin ulceration (breakdown) and nearly always occurs over a bony prominence. Remember though, some discolourations and apparent abnormalities such as birthmarks and moles are present at birth (congenital) and do not represent a specific problem or disorder. Be sensitive to how your patient may feel about the presence of these, particularly if they are highly visible.

Texture

Assessing skin texture by visual (and touch) examination will reveal factors such as whether the skin is rough, smooth, bumpy, papery or thickened. Rough skin on the foot, for example, could be due to excessive dryness as a result of diabetic neuropathy; smooth, hairless skin on the lower leg could be secondary to arterial disease; bumpy skin may be due to cold (remember what the arrector pili muscle does?); papery, thin skin may be due to long-term use of steroids and thickened skin on the hands or feet could be due to callus formation (an excess build-up of epidermal cells in response to prolonged friction).

Elasticity

A loss of elasticity can indicate advancing age or a more significant problem such as dehydration. Well-elasticised and hydrated skin springs back into place easily, while poorly elasticised or dehydrated skin sinks back slowly. The ability of the skin to spring back into shape is known as skin turgor.

Activity 7.12

Assess your skin turgor. Using your thumb and first finger, gently lift the skin on the back of your hand for a few seconds then let it fall naturally back into place. Make a note of what happened.

Temperature

Skin should be warm to touch. Extremes of temperature, for example, the skin is too hot or too cold, can indicate a whole range of underlying problems such as infection, hormonal imbalance or hypothermia. Skin temperature can initially be assessed by laying the back of your hand over an area of the skin and judging how warm or cool the skin feels compared to your own. This is what is called a subjective assessment; in other words, it is based on opinion rather than fact.

Integrity

Skin should always be assessed for integrity, that is, Is it all in one piece? A break in the continuity of the skin is known as a wound. Wounds can be very distressing for patients; they can cause pain (Wulf and Baron, 2004), smell (Haughton and Young, 2007) and wetness (Vuolo, 2004) and they may affect the patients' body image and therefore self-esteem (Dealey, 2005). A wound in the skin can also affect the skins' normal function (see Section '**Functions of the skin**') in different ways depending on the size of the wound and the type of the wound. Any wound provides an entrance into the body which can be used by microorganisms to cause infection or disease; large wounds where there are significant areas of skin loss may result in decreased vitamin D synthesis; highly exuding wounds can result in large amounts of fluid loss.

All skin assessments should be carried out in private as quietly and discreetly as possible, for example, make sure you cannot be overheard, and make sure you are not interrupted. A warm room and good lighting are essential (Lawton, 1998), as is a blanket (Peters, 2001).

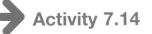

Activity 7.13

Why do you think the following are essential when carrying out a full skin assessment?

(a) A warm room
(b) Good lighting
(c) A blanket

Skin care

Keeping the skin clean and dry is an essential nursing skill. Good skin care prevents the build-up of dirt and moisture and the development of unpleasant body odour. Skin care usually involves washing and drying the skin and may include the use of additional products such as moisturisers and deodorisers.

Explaining why you want to cleanse the skin will help your patients understand what you want to do whilst giving them the opportunity to care for their own skin hygiene helps maintain their independence as well as raising self-esteem. Do remember that routines and preferences can vary considerably according to cultural, religious and personal beliefs, so it is important to work with your patient to find a routine that works for both of you.

Activity 7.14

1. Check your bathroom cabinet; how many different hygiene products can you find?
2. Which one would you want to take with you if you were admitted to hospital?
3. Why do you think it is important to ask the patients about their personal preferences when choosing hygiene products for them?

Make a note of your answers here.

What to use?

The range of skin cleansing products on offer is huge and includes traditional bar soaps, shower gels, soaps with added moisturisers, liquid soaps and soap substitutes.

Traditional bar soaps

These tend to have a high alkalinity (some as high as 9.0) which alters the natural pH of the skin, breaking down the protective acid mantle and stripping it of its surface moisture (lipids). The result can be dry, cracked and reddened skin. Once the skin's healthy balance has been altered in this way, it is vulnerable to breakdown and damage, particularly in the older population (Cooper and Gray, 2001). It is not certain if pH-balanced soaps are necessary but soaps with a pH closer to that of the skin (5.4–5.9) are certainly the better option. The modern synthetic detergents or 'syndets' offer additional benefits such as bacterial regulating properties (through pH balance) and high tolerance profiles, which are particularly useful for patients with skin diseases such as acne vulgaris and contact dermatitis as well as being of value for healthy skin types (Schmid and Korting, 2006).

Shower gels and liquid soaps

With easy to use pump or squeeze bottle dispensers, these soaps (often syndets) are convenient and practical; although the ingredients will not necessarily be any more or less harsh than those of traditional soap bars.

Soap substitutes or alternatives

Many of these cleanse the skin gently and have an additional moisturising element which leaves the skin feeling soft after washing. Aqueous cream BP is commonly used for this purpose as it is readily available from any pharmacy and is relatively cheap compared with branded products. Foam skin cleansers such as Clinisan® also make suitable alternatives to traditional soaps providing gentle but effective cleansing, particularly after episodes of incontinence (Cooper and Gray, 2001),

How should skin be cleansed?

Skin care should take place in private and without interruption. Before removing your patient's clothing, ensure that you have all the equipment you require and that the room temperature is comfortable. When you have decided what to use, apply the cleansing product according to the manufacturers' instructions. If the product has to be removed, for example bar soap and shower gel, it should be washed off with warm water and a soft disposable cloth. If the patients wish to use their own flannel/cloth, you will need to ensure it is washed regularly to keep it clean and smelling fresh.

When to cleanse?

The frequency of washing is a matter of personal choice but many people like to have a 'strip' wash, shower or bath at least once per day, perhaps more often in hot weather. Discuss your patients' preferences with them and record them for other member of the team to see. It is also necessary to cleanse the skin after any episodes of urinary or faecal incontinence and after contact with body fluids such as vomit or blood. Patients are also usually grateful for an extra wash when they are sweating profusely.

How should skin be dried?

The skin should be gently patted dry with a clean, soft towel. Drying the skin properly is very important but vigorous rubbing is unnecessary; it can cause patient discomfort and skin damage.

The use of talcum powder is not advocated; it has a tendency to build up between uses leading to pore clogging and skin maceration and can affect the performance of disposable incontinence pads (Le Lievre, 2000). It has also been suggested that talcum powder moistened with sweat or urine can lead to encrustations which can cause skin damage or breakdown (Benbow, 2001). The perfumes in some talcum powders may also be problematic for patients with sensitive skins.

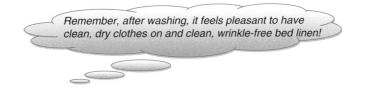

Remember, after washing, it feels pleasant to have clean, dry clothes on and clean, wrinkle-free bed linen!

Managing the incontinent patient's skin

Earlier in this chapter, the skin's pH was noted to be between 5.4 and 5.9 (Schmid and Korting, 2006); this pH range denotes a slightly acidic environment. However, urine and faeces are both alkaline in nature and therefore when they come into contact with the skin they disturb the normal pH balance. The alteration in skin pH can result in destruction of the skins' normal protective mantle. Urine and faeces combined can cause skin irritation which can progress to dermatitis excoriation (Fiers, 1996); a red, painful, inflammation of the skin which can extend to blistering and skin breakdown. Excess moisture on the skin combined with enzyme and bacterial activity can also result in the breakdown of vulnerable skin (Wounds UK, 2006) as can the use of ordinary soap and water. For these patients, foams cleansers tend to be an effective but skin-friendly alternative. Skin should therefore be cleansed and dried after every episode of incontinence. After drying, the skin can be partially protected from contact with urine or faeces by the use of a barrier cream or ointment. These should be applied and re-applied according to the manufacturer's instructions.

Common skin problems

During skin care is the ideal time to talk with your patients and discuss any worries or concerns they may have. It is also an ideal opportunity to examine their skin for any problems. If you observe anything that is unusual or problematic, ensure that you record your findings and communicate them to an appropriately qualified colleague.

Activity 7.15

Take a moment to reflect on your clinical experience.
What kind of skin conditions or problems have you encountered?
How were they managed?
What effect did they have on the patient?
How will these experiences influence the way that you will manage the same or similar situations in the future?

Write down your reflections here.

Some of the more common skin problems you may come across are pressure damage, dryness, maceration, skin tears and wounds.

Pressure damage

A pressure ulcer is an area of localised damage to the skin and underlying tissue caused by pressure, shear, and friction, or a combination of these (European Pressure Ulcer Advisory Panel, 1998). When the skin is subjected to these external forces, the blood supply to the skin is reduced or stopped completely resulting in tissue (skin) damage or skin death. This can be seen externally as patches of permanent discolouration, blistering or ulceration of the skin (see Figure 7.1). Extensive pressure damage can extend right through the skin layers and affect muscle, nerves and tendon too; bone may be exposed in the most severe cases (see Figure 7.1).

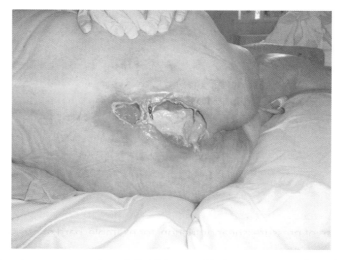

Figure 7.1   Extensive pressure ulcer: full thickness skin loss, nerve and tendon involvement.

Pressure ulcers can be distressing and painful for patients. They can result in decreased mobility, increased length of illness and a prolonged hospital stay. They also cost a great deal of money to treat with costs incurred by elements of care such as dressings, staff time, equipment, theatre time and pharmaceuticals. Preventing pressure damage is therefore very important, and whilst it is not solely the responsibility of the nurse, it is certainly an essential element of good nursing care.

Activity 7.16

Try this experiment: Cross your legs at the knee for 60 s. Now uncross them and look at the knee underneath. You may have noticed the skin initially looking pale (blanched) then quickly becoming flushed (reddened). **Note:** These skin changes are more difficult to see in darkly pigmented skin, so you will need to observe the affected area carefully.

What causes these changes?
When your legs were crossed you were applying pressure to the skin and the underlying bone. The pressure was squeezing closed the small blood vessels in the skin so that the blood flow was slowed right down; the reduction in blood flow to the area resulted in the pale or blanched appearance of the skin. When you uncrossed your legs, that is, took the pressure off, the small blood vessels opened up again and the blood flowed back into the area. In fact, the body probably rushed in some extra blood to compensate for the previous reduction in blood flow. This resulted in the temporary flushing or reddening that you saw.

The extra rush of blood to the skin after a period of blood flow reduction is a normal physiological response intended to prevent any permanent skin damage happening. This response is called reactive hyperaemia.

Unfortunately, reactive hyperaemia can only compensate for a temporary loss of blood flow. For some patients, this simply isn't enough. The skin is an organ just like the brain and the liver and it needs a constant supply of blood to survive. Therefore, if pressure reduces or stops blood flow for long, enough skin damage or death will occur. For some patients, the problems arise because the body cannot supply enough well-oxygenated blood to the skin even when the pressure stopping the blood flow has been removed; this may be because of conditions such as chronic cardiac failure or chronic respiratory disease. Whatever the cause, once pressure damage has occurred it is irreversible.

What can you do?

- Know which patients are at risk of developing pressure damage.
- Ensure the skin is well nourished and hydrated.
- Remove any cause of pressure, shear or friction, for example, hard mattress, poor seating.
- Encourage your patients to move around independently to improve the circulation (blood supply) to their skin.

- If your patients are unable to move then re-position them regularly.
- Handle the skin carefully; avoid any dragging or tearing of skin tissues.
- Keep the skin clean and dry, especially after episodes of incontinence.

"But how will I know if my patient is at risk of developing pressure damage?"

Anybody who is sitting or lying in one position for a period of time, particularly if it is on a hard surface, could develop pressure damage. They are also at risk if they are sliding down on a bed or chair surface. Other risk factors include conditions that affect the supply or quality of blood flow, for example paraplaegia, diabetes. Nobody knows how long it takes to develop pressure damage but it can happen very quickly.

It is more likely if:

- The person's skin is in poor condition; this results in the skin being less tolerant to pressure.
- The person is unable to move independently, that is, he or she is immobile. This means the person cannot move to allow the blood supply back into the area of skin that is being starved of it.
- The person cannot sense the need to change position. Normally, the nerves in the skin sense when we have been in one position for too long and the skin is being starved of blood. A message is sent to the brain to tell us to move and allow the blood back in, which revives the skin. This safety mechanism even works when we are asleep.

In Activity 7.17 try to think of three causes of each. This will give you some idea of who might be at risk of pressure damage.

Activity 7.17

Increased risk of pressure damage	Cause
Poor skin condition	1. 2. 3.
Immobility	1. 2. 3.
Lack of sensation	1. 2. 3.

Warning!

The onset of pressure damage may be reported as a sensation of numbness, tingling or pain. It may be seen as a patch of permanent redness (erythema) which does not turn white (blanch) when you apply light finger pressure. It may be felt as an area of hardened or oedematous skin. If you think your patient is at risk or if you notice any of the above warning signs, please ensure you report it to a senior member of the nursing team and document your findings clearly.

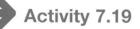

Activity 7.18

Take a moment to reflect on your clinical experience.
Have you nursed anybody at risk of pressure damage?
Have you nursed anyone with existing pressure damage?
What measures were used to protect their skin?
How will your nursing practice change now that you know more about who is at risk of pressure damage?

Write down your reflections in a notebook and keep for future reference.

Wounds

A wound is a break in the continuity of the skin. Pressure ulcers (previously known as pressure sores, bed sores or decubitus ulcers) are wounds and so are leg ulcers and burns. What other kinds of wounds have you seen?

Activity 7.19

Make a list of all the other types of wounds you have seen.

Wounds are sometimes classified according to the depth as well as the type. The depth of a wound may be described as superficial, partial thickness or full thickness. These terms refer to the level of skin damage that has occurred as a result of the wound.

➤ Activity 7.20

Use your Nurses' dictionary to find out the exact meaning of the terms superficial, partial thickness and full thickness.

Superficial: ....

Partial thickness: ....

Full thickness: ....

Now think about the wounds you have seen in clinical practice and decide which description best matches each. Make a note of your findings here.

Wounds are also described by their size, colour, smell, wetness (exudate), infection status and position on the body. All these factors (and more) will tell you something about the wound you are looking at and how it is best treated. However, decisions about the care of wounds must be made by a qualified healthcare professional who has recent experience and knowledge of the management of wounds. You may find it helpful to ask your mentor to explain the wound assessment and management process the next time you see a patient with a wound in clinical practice.

Skin tears

Skin tears are wounds that tend to happen when the skin is papery and thin; therefore, it is often the elderly who are at risk. They happen easily, when a leg or arm is accidentally knocked the skin layers tear apart revealing an open wound (see Figure 7.2).

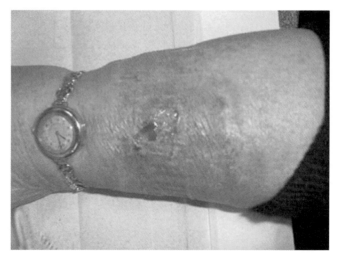

Figure 7.2   Skin tear on arm

What can you do?

- Know who is at risk, for example older people, people on long-term steroid therapy.
- Be aware of vulnerable areas such as the front of the leg, back of hand or arm.
- Handle skin carefully, for example, do not drag at the skin and pat dry with soft towel after washing.
- Avoid using sticky tapes or plasters on the skin.
- Use clothing to add protection if appropriate, for example long trousers to cover up the lower leg.

Dryness

As discussed earlier, dry skin is caused by a number of factors such as the ageing process, environment, dehydration and underlying disease. The repeated use of soap also strips the skin of its natural coating of protective lipids leading to further dryness.

What can you do?

- Use soap substitutes or emulsifying ointments, for example Oilatum® or E45®.
- Dry skin carefully by patting with soft towel.
- Apply bland, non-perfumed moisturisers, for example 50/50 white soft and liquid paraffin.
- Encourage an adequate intake of fluid.
- Regulate the room temperature and use a humidifier to add moisture to the air.

Oedema

Oedema is the build-up of fluid in the spaces between the cells of the skin tissue. It has numerous causes including malnutrition, congestive cardiac failure and infection. Oedematous skin can feel spongy and/or fairly firm depending on the amount of fluid present. Sometimes it is possible to feel the fluid on gentle handling of the skin and there may be pitting marks left on the skin when it is gently pressed.

What can you do?

- Be aware of vulnerable areas, for example, where tissue fluid has accumulated.
- Handle the skin carefully especially when washing, changing clothes and re-positioning.
- Pat skin dry with soft towel after washing.
- Avoid using sticky tapes or plasters on the skin.

Maceration

Maceration has been defined as the softening and breaking down of skin resulting from prolonged exposure to moisture (Cutting and White, 2002).

Common sources of moisture include sweat, urinary incontinence, wound fluid (exudate) or natural fluid loss through the surface of the skin (trans-epidermal water loss or TEWL for short). The moisture sits on the skin and re-hydrates the flattened, dry epidermal cells of the stratum corneum. As these cells become plump with moisture, the skin turns pale and feels soft/spongy. This spongy, overly moist skin is very vulnerable to damage (see Figure 7.3).

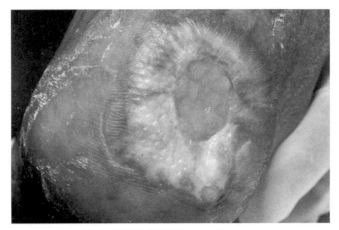

Figure 7.3   Macerated skin surrounding a pressure ulcer

What can you do?

- Know who are at risk, for example, patients with wet wounds, patients who are incontinent, patients who are sweating profusely.
- Keep skin clean and dry, especially after episodes of incontinence.
- Use a skin protectanct such as Cavilon® when exposure to moisture is unavoidable.
- Avoid soaking skin in water for long periods, for example soaking legs and feet.

On completion of this chapter, you should have a good understanding of the skin and of the key principles of skin care. You should also be able to demonstrate an awareness of commonly encountered skin-related problems. To check your understanding, work your way through the following checklist:

Aspect of care	Yes or no?
Can you describe the anatomical structure of the skin?	
Can you identify the core functions of the skin?	
Do you know how to care for the skin?	
Do you know about some of the more common skin-related problems?	
Are you able to explain why good skin care is one of the key elements of essential nursing care?	
Can you give examples of how the key themes of communication, privacy and dignity and health and safety, relate to the principles of good skin care?	

> **Activity 7.21**
>
> Now reflect on your clinical placement experiences.
>
> What happened?
>
> How did it make you feel?
>
> What would you do differently (if anything) next time?

Chapter summary

This chapter discusses many important aspects of skin and skin care starting with skin anatomy and function, working through to assessment and then on to prevention and management of skin damage. It has highlighted the importance of understanding how the skin works in order to make effective decisions about how best to care for it. Now you have completed the chapter, you should now feel confident in your ability to plan effective skin care for your clients or patients. Remember, skin care is one of the most fundamental aspects of nursing care and something that every nurse should be proud to do well.

Answers to Activities

Activity 7.1 Key terms

Use your nursing dictionary to complete the glossary below; this is good preparation for reading the rest of the chapter.

Term	Definition
Abrasion	Superficial graze
Arrector pili	The small muscle found at the base of the hair strand which connects the hair follicle to the dermis
Callus	An area of skin which has become relatively thick and hard in response to repeated contact or pressure
Capillary	A minute blood vessel which connects arteriole and venule
Carotene	An orange/yellow pigment
Chloracne	An acne-like skin disorder which can develop after prolonged exposure to chlorinated hydrocarbons
Connective tissue	Tissue that forms the supporting and connecting structures of the body
Epidermis	The uppermost (outer) layer of the skin
Dermis	The lower layer of skin, for example, that lies beneath the epidermis
Diabetic neuropathy	A disease or abnormality of the nervous system
Haemoglobin	An iron containing protein which transports oxygen in the blood
Hypodermis	A layer of cells that secretes chitin
Irritant contact dermatitis	Skin inflammation which arises following contact with an irritating substance or allergen
Keratinocytes	An epidermal cell that produces keratin
Laceration	A jagged wound or cut
Lipid	A water insoluble, fat-like substance
Melanin	A dark coloured pigment
Microorganism	An organism that can only be seen with a microscope, for example, bacteria, fungi
Oedema	An abnormal accumulation of fluid in the tissue spaces
Pigment	A colouring matter
Puncture wound	A wound produced by a narrow, pointed object

Activity 7.1 (*Continued*)

Sebaceous glands	A gland in the dermis that produces and secrete sebum
Sebum	Oily secretion of the sebaceous gland, contains fat, keratin and cellular debris
Shearing force	Applied force resulting in distortion of the skin tissues
Stratum basale	Deepest layer of the epidermis
Stratum corneum	Outer (horny) layer of the epidermis
Stratum granulosum	Epidermal layer between lucidum and spinosum
Stratum lucidum	Epidermal layer beneath corneum
Stratum spinosum	Epidermal layer between granulosum and basale
Sudoriferous glands	Sweat producing gland
Tensile strength	Ability to withstand stretching or straining
Turgor	Normal tension or fullness
Vasoconstriction	Narrowing of blood vessel
Vasodilation	Widening of blood vessel

Activity 7.2

Name the different layers of the epidermis.
The different layers of the epidermis are:
1. stratum basale
2. stratum spinosum
3. stratum granulosum
4. stratum lucidum (thick skin only)
5. stratum corneum

Activity 7.3

Where on the body do you think you might find *thin* skin?
Thin (hairy) skin covers all parts of the body except the palms (including the palmar surface of the fingers) and the soles of the feet.

Where on the body do you think you might find *thick* skin?
The palms of the hands, palmar surface of the fingers and the soles of the feet are covered by thick (hairless) skin.

Activity 7.4

Can you accurately label this diagram of the skin?

The skin diagram should be labelled as followed:

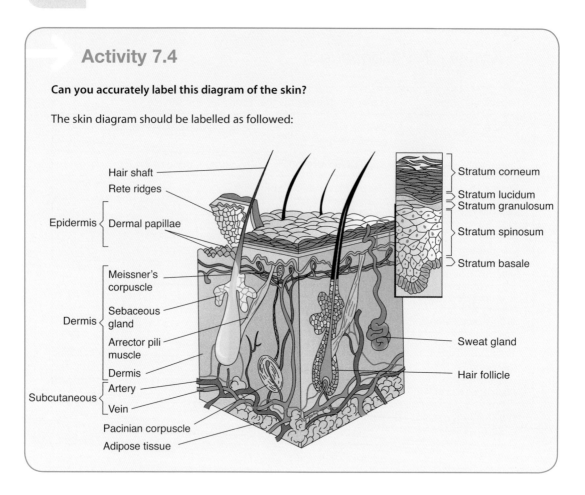

Activity 7.5

Think about tensile strength. List three examples of when skin might be subjected to a pulling force.

You could have included:

1. Going down a slide
2. Pulling somebody up by the hand
3. The stretching of skin experienced during advanced pregnancy

Activity 7.6

Find out the definitions of each of the six blood cooling mechanisms.

Mechanism	Definition
Radiation	The transfer of heat from one object to another without actual contact. The body radiates heat to every object near it, that's why lots of people standing very close together get very hot!
Conduction	The transfer of heat from one object to another through contact. Heat will always transfer to the cooler of the two objects. If you place a hand on a cool marble surface some of your body warmth will be transferred to the marble.
Convection	The transfer of heat from the body to air which then rises to be replaced by cooler air which is also then heated. Wrapping up warmly in the cold weather stops loss of heat by convection, whilst reducing in layers in the warm weather helps to keep you cool.
Evaporation	Sweat is continuously evaporated from the surface of the skin. This keeps the body cool unless the air is very moist (humid) already, in which case evaporation cannot occur. The result is often a continual drip of sweat — yuk!
Respiration	Body heat is lost through water vapour which evaporates when we breathe out.
Excretion	A small amount of body heat is lost through the passage of urine and faeces.

Activity 7.7

Watch how the fine hairs on your arm respond to very cold and very warm temperatures.
You should have seen the fine hairs on your arm lie flat when you were feeling very warm and stand upright when you were feeling very cold.

Activity 7.8

Look at your face in the mirror. What words would you use to describe your skin?
You may have used words to describe: colour (black, creamy, flushed); texture (rough, smooth, pitted, scarred); health (vibrant, dull, blooming); or age (young, old, wrinkled).

Activity 7.9

List three indoor (internal) occupations which may affect skin health.

1. Chef/cook
2. Office worker
3. Factory worker

List three outdoor (external) occupations which may affect skin health.

1. Fisherman
2. Farmer
3. Fire fighter

Activity 7.10

Make a list of people who you think could be at risk of malnutrition.

You may have included:

1. Patients with an illness or disease affecting their ability to eat or drink
2. Patients who have just had surgery
3. Intravenous drug users
4. People with psychological disorders such as bulimia or anorexia nervosa
5. People on low incomes
6. People who are socially isolated
7. The elderly
8. The immobile

Activity 7.11

Air conditioning?	Turn it down or off when not needed
Central heating?	Turn it down or off when not needed. Use a humidifier to improve air moisture content.
Smoking?	Avoid smoking areas. Use good extractor/ventilation systems. Open windows.
Sun exposure?	Use UV protection suntan lotion, wear hat, sunglasses. Stay out of midday sun. Drink plenty of non-alcoholic fluids.
Poor nutrition?	Encourage a diet with all the essential nutrients necessary for skin and total body health.
Poor hydration?	Encourage 6–8 cups of fluid per day per adult.

Activity 7.12

Assess your skin turgor. Using your thumb and first finger, gently lift the skin on the back of your hand for a few seconds then let it fall naturally back into place. Make a note of what happened.

Your observations should reflect what you have read about the skin turgor. Keep the record of your findings and check again in a year's time; see if there is any difference!

Activity 7.13

Why do you think the following are essential when carrying out a full skin assessment?

(a) **A warm room** is necessary because extreme temperatures affect skin colour and you will need to see the skin at its normal colour to assess it accurately.
(b) **Good lighting** is necessary to see the skin clearly.
(c) **A blanket** must be used to ensure patient modesty is maintained. This is important at all times but particularly when examining 'private' areas such as the genitals or breasts.

Well done if you thought of some other reasons too.

Activity 7.14

1. **Check your bathroom cabinet; how many different hygiene products can you find?**
2. **Which one would you want to take with you if you were admitted to hospital?**
3. **Why do you think it is important to ask the patients about their personal preferences when choosing hygiene products for them?**

Make a note of your answers here.
You may have found many different products or just a few. What you have will depend on many different factors such as price, effectiveness, packaging, smell, availability, environmental impact or animal testing. Your choice of what to take to hospital may also depend on product size, storage space and access to washing facilities. How will you use this knowledge next time you care for a patient's hygiene needs?

Activity 7.15

Reflection

Activity 7.16

Experiment

Activity 7.17

Increased risk of pressure damage	Cause
Poor skin condition	1. Age 2. Disease, for example cancer, diabetes 3. Medication, for example steroids, malnutrition, oedema, incontinence
Immobility	1. Paralysis 2. Arthritis 3. Broken limb
Lack of sensation	1. Loss of consciousness 2. Some drugs, for example anaesthetics, analgesics 3. Nerve damage, for example neuropathy, stroke

Activity 7.18

Reflection

Activity 7.19

Make a list of all the other types of wounds you have seen.
Here are some of the wound types you may have seen: surgical wound, laceration, abrasion, malignant wound, self-inflicted wound, diabetic ulcer, puncture wound, animal or insect bite.

Activity 7.20

Use your Nurses' dictionary to find out the exact meaning of the terms superficial, partial thickness and full thickness.
Superficial: skin damage or injury affecting the surface only, that is, the epidermis
Partial thickness: skin damage or injury affecting the epidermis and part of the dermis too
Full thickness: skin damage or injury affecting the epidermis and extending all the way through the dermis
Now think about the wounds you have seen in clinical practice and decide which description best matches each. Make a note of your findings.

Activity 7.21

Now reflect on your clinical experiences of caring for the skin care needs of a patient. Write what happened, how it made you feel and what would you do differently (if anything) next time when caring for a patient with skin care needs.

This is your personal experience of caring for a patient with some common skin-related problems. Reflect your own personal feelings in relation to your learning needs. You may have more than one learning need; hence, you could use the same subheadings to address the issues.

What happened?
● Describe the scenario briefly relating to your learning need.

How did it make you feel?
● Did you feel good or bad about it?
● Did you have adequate underpinning knowledge to carry out the care?
● If you had previous experience of a similar situation, was it useful this time?

What would you do differently (if anything) next time?
● Has this personal experience encouraged you to do further reading and gain more practice under supervision?

This is only a guide. Please address the subheadings to meet your own learning needs.

References

Baranoski, S. and Ayello, E.A. (2004) *Wound Care Essentials. Practice Principles* (New York: Springhouse).

Benbow, M. (2001) Readers' questions: use of talcum powder. *Journal of Wound Care* **10** (2), 22.

British Nutrition Foundation (2003) Nutrition basics: Healthy Eating. http://www.britishnutrition.org.uk/home.asp?siteId=43&sectionId=320&parentSection=299&which=1 (accessed 26 May 2007).

Cooper, P. and Gray, D. (2001) Comparison of two skin care regimes for incontinence. *British Journal of Nursing (Suppl.)* **10** (6), 6–20.

Cua, A.B., Wilhelm, K.-P. and Maibach, H.I. (1990) Elastic properties of skin: in relation to age, sex and anatomical region. *Archives of Dermatological Research* **282** (5), 283–288.

Cutting, K. and White, R.J. (2002) Maceration of the skin and the wound bed. 1: Its nature and causes. *Journal of Wound Care* **11** (7), 275–278.

Dealey, C. (2005) *The Care of Wounds: A Guide for Nurses*, 3rd edn (Oxford: Blackwell Publishing).

English, J.S., Dawe, R.S. and Ferguson, J. (2003) Environmental effects and skin disease. *British Medical Bulletin* **68** (1), 129–142.

European Pressure Ulcer Advisory Panel (1998) Pressure ulcer treatment guidelines. http://www.epuap.org/gltreatment.html (accessed 25 May 2007).

Fiers, S.A. (1996) Breaking the cycle: the etiology of incontinence dermatitis and evaluating and using skin care products. *Ostomy/Wound Management* **42** (3), 32–34, 36, 38–40.

Haughton, W. and Young, T. (2007) Common problems in wound care: malodorous wounds. *British Journal of Nursing* **4** (16), 959–963.

Hughes, E. (2001) Skin: its structure and function and related pathology. In *Dermatology Nursing: A Practical Guide*, E. Hughes and J. Van Onselen, eds (London: Harcourt), pp. 1–18.

Jenkins, G.W., Kemnitz, C.P. and Tortora, G.J. (2007) *Anatomy and Physiology: From Science to Life* (West Sussex: Wiley).

Knight, S. (2003) *Muscles, Bones and Skin*, 2nd edn (Oxford: Elsevier Science).

Lawton, S. (1998) Assessing the skin. *Professional Nurse* **13** (4), S5–S7.

Le Lievre, S.E. (2000) Care of the incontinent client's skin. *Journal of Community Nursing* **14** (2), 26–32.

Leung, W.C. and Harvey, I. (2002) Is skin ageing in the elderly caused by sun exposure or smoking? *British Journal of Dermatology* **147** (6), 1187–1191.

National Prescribing Centre (1998) Oral nutritional support. *MeRecC Bulletin (Part 1)* **9** (7) 25.

Perfect, H., Wilson, H. and Garabaldinos, T. (2001) Phototherapy. In *Dermatology Nursing: A Practical Guide*, E. Hughes and J. Van Onselen, eds (London: Harcourt), pp. 65–79.

Peters, J. (2001) Assessment of the dermatology patient. In *Dermatology Nursing: A Practical Guide*, E. Hughes and J. Van Onselen, eds (London: Harcourt), pp. 19–39.

Schmid, M.H. and Korting, H.C. (1995) The concept of the acid mantle of the skin: its relevance for the choice of skin cleansers. *Dermatology* **191** (4), 276–280.

Schmid, M.-H. and Korting, H.C. (2006) The pH of the skin surface and its' impact on the barrier function. *Skin Pharmacology and Physiology* **19** (6), 296–302.

Tur, E., Yosipovitvh, G. and Oren-Vulfs, S. (1992) Chronic and acute effects of cigarette smoking on skin blood flow. *Angiology* **43** (4), 328–335.

Watson, R. (2000) *Anatomy and Physiology for Nurses*, 11th edn (Oxford: Elsevier Science).

Waeber, B., Schaller, M.D., Nussberger, J., Bussien, J.P., Hofbauer, K.G. and Brunner, H.R. (1984) Skin blood flow reduction induced by cigarette smoking: role of vasopressin. *American Journal of Physiology — Heart and Circulatory Physiology* **247** (6), H895–H901.

Wounds UK (2006) *Best Practice Statement: Care of the Older Person's Skin* (Aberdeen: Wounds UK).

Vuolo, J. (2004) Current options for managing the problem of excess wound exudate. *Professional Nurse* **19** (9), 487–491.

Wulf, H. and Baron, R. (2004) The theory of pain. In *Pain at Wound Dressing Changes – A EWMA Position Document*. (London: MEP).

Further reading

Clark, M. (2004) *Pressure Ulcers: Recent Advances in Tissue Viability* (London: Quay Books).

Dealey, C. (2005) *The Care of Wounds: A Guide for Nurses*, 3rd edn (Oxford: Blackwell).

Ritchie, J. (2007) *Crash Course: Muscles, Bones and Skin*, 3rd edn (Oxford: Mosby (Elsevier)).

Waugh, A. and Grant, A. (2001) *Ross and Wilson Anatomy and Physiology in Health and Illness*, 10th edn (London: Churchill Livingstone).

Wounds UK (2006) *Best Practice Statement: Care of the Older Person's Skin* (Aberdeen: Wounds UK).

Useful websites

British Association for Parenteral and Enteral Nutrition (BAPEN) — http://www.bapen.org.uk/

European Pressure Ulcer Advisory Panel — www.epuap.org/

National Eczema Society — www.eczema.org/

National Institute of Clinical Excellence — www.nice.org.uk/

NHS Direct — www.nhsdirect.nhs.uk/

Skin Care Campaign — www.skincarecampaign.org/

World Wide Wounds website — www.worldwidewounds.com/

Principles of first aid

LOUISE LAWSON

Aims

The aim of this chapter is to introduce you to the key principles of first aid and provide with an overview of the sequence of priorities in a first aid situation and how to deal with some common emergencies.

Learning objectives

On completion of this chapter, you will learn to:
- Recognise the priorities in a first aid situation in any environment
- Identify essential skills in basic life support
- Demonstrate an awareness of some common emergencies
- Complete the activities in order to prepare you for situations outside or in clinical placements

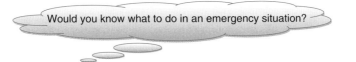

Would you know what to do in an emergency situation?

Introduction

First aid is the initial emergency care given immediately upon arrival at the scene to an ill or injured person (St John Ambulance *et al.*, 2006) and continues until professional medical assistance takes over the care of the casualty. During your nursing programme, you may undergo training in basic life support in a simulated environment that is intended for use in the clinical area. However, you may be exposed to a situation where you will not have the benefit of a team of experts who can help you. You may have only experienced emergencies in a hospital environment and this can be stressful for anyone. Even experienced healthcare practitioners can feel nervous in a first aid scenario despite having the training, expertise and skills. Wardrope and Mackenzie (2004) have suggested that emergency situations cause stress, especially if they are unfamiliar or present new and different challenges.

You do not need to study a first aid course to be able to save a life; however, the principles of first aid do not take long to learn. It can be very frightening when dealing with someone who has collapsed or is choking, and no book or manual will be able to prepare you for a real-life situation, whether in the clinical area or in the supermarket. However, you must remember that as hard as you try, some casualties do not respond to treatment and may die, though any attempt at saving someone is better than nothing. When you become a qualified nurse, you will have a duty of care to attend to any emergency situation; however, the law does not require lay people to volunteer help, unless there is a pre-existing duty, such as a healthcare professional like yourself (Dimond, 2008). However, Dimond (2005) highlighted that it does not matter whether the healthcare professional is in uniform, unless the uniform signifies that you are on duty.

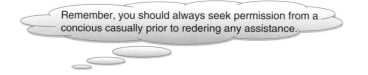

Remember, you should always seek permission from a concious casually prior to redering any assistance.

Once you begin to give assistance, you have a responsibility to provide first aid in accordance with your level of training and competence.

The Nursing and Midwifery Council (NMC) stated in the previous Code of Professional Conduct (NMC, 2004 *clause 8.5*) that '*in an emergency, in or outside the work setting, you have a professional duty to provide care. The care provided would be judged against what could be reasonably expected from someone with your knowledge, skills and abilities when placed in those particular circumstances.*' This heightened the debate for nurses to have a greater knowledge of first aid (McBean, 2002). The Code however (NMC, 2008) states '*You must have the knowledge and skills for safe and effective practice when working without direct supervision and that you must recognise and work within the limits of your competence*'. Therefore, any nurse claiming to have the professional nursing skills must use those skills at an ordinary competent level when exercising the art of nursing both in and out of the hospital environment (Ford *et al.*, 2000). The Resuscitation Council (2008) state that healthcare institutions have an obligation to provide an effective resuscitation service and to ensure that all staff receive training and regular updates for maintaining a level of competence appropriate to each individual's employed role. Therefore, the principles of first aid and basic life support training are included as part of the pre-registration curriculum, though these tend to focus on basic life support in a hospital environment, but neglect to pass on skills which could save a life on the street (BBC, 1999). These skills should be kept up to date on an annual basis as part of your mandatory training.

This chapter will focus on the primary assessment and the principles of basic life support such as cardio-pulmonary resuscitation (CPR); however, it is not intended to replace any formal first aid instruction. It will also consider choking, shock and fractures. By completing this chapter, it should provide you with an overview of these common emergencies whether in or out of the hospital environment in any situation. The focus of this chapter will be based on the adult patient/casualty and will be based on the resuscitation guidelines of the Resuscitation Council UK (2005a). The chapter is intended to offer an insight into some emergency situations and provide you with enough information needed for those first vital moments. For the purpose of this chapter, the patient will be referred to as the 'casualty'.

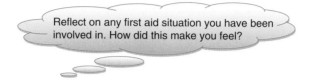

Reflect on any first aid situation you have been involved in. How did this make you feel?

The first aid kit

We all take certain measures to prevent accidents but despite our best efforts, emergencies may arise. You may be in a situation in or outside of the clinical area when an accident takes place, so best to be prepared. Besides a well-stocked and functional first aid kit, preparation is the most important tool you can have at your disposal and prevention is better than cure. You can use your first aid kit at home or keep in the car to help you deal with minor injuries or to keep major injuries stable until help arrives. There are minimum standards in what to put in a first aid kit; however, the contents may be dependent on the situation or environment. You should not keep tablets or medicines in a first aid box.

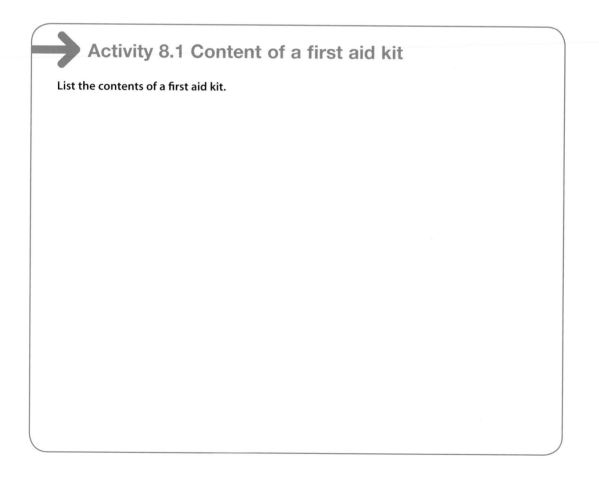

Activity 8.1 Content of a first aid kit

List the contents of a first aid kit.

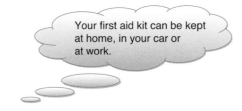

Your first aid kit can be kept at home, in your car or at work.

Activity 8.2 First aid containers

What do you think should be the golden rules for first aid containers?

Your priorities in a first aid situation

Your priorities in any first aid situation are to:

- Preserve life if possible
- Protect the casualty, yourself and any bystanders
- Promote recovery

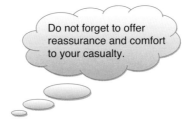

Do not forget to offer reassurance and comfort to your casualty.

- Call for help
- Assess the situation
- Give appropriate treatment
- Monitor the casualty for any changes in condition (Sevett, 2006)

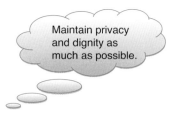

Maintain privacy and dignity as much as possible.

A fundamental knowledge of first aid can enable the nurse to administer confidently, competently and safely what could be a life-saving action (Dean, 2005). However, it is important to remember the golden rule, 'first do no harm, whilst applying the term calculated risk' (St John Ambulance *et al.*, 2006).

First of all, it is essential that you look for signs of **Danger**. Look around you and, in particular, look upwards if a patient is on the floor as something may have fallen from above. Look for other hazards such as live wires, fire, or consider oncoming traffic is not a danger to you or your casualty. Do not attempt to be a hero; you cannot help your casualties if you are injured too. It is important to stay calm as you may notice that your heart is beating faster and you may be sweating. This is in response to the release of hormones as the 'fight or flight' response occurs.

Check the casualty' level of **Response** to assess consciousness. Before you start any rescue efforts, you must remember to check the casualty for responsiveness. If you suspect that the casualty has sustained spinal or neck injury, do not move or shake him or her. Does the casualty respond to sound, touch or pain? Give a verbal command — 'hello, can you hear me — can you open your eyes?' — speak loudly and clear. Assess the casualty's level of response using the acronym AVPU code. This stands for:

- **A** — is the casualty alert?
- **V** — does the casualty respond to voice?
- **P** — does the casualty respond to pain?
- **U** — is the casualty unresponsive to stimulus (St John Ambulance *et al.*, 2006)?

If someone besides you is present, one should dial 999 immediately. If you are alone with the casualty, try to **Shout** for help prior to starting CPR. In the practice setting, help should be available almost immediately, so if you are in an environment that does not have this sort of assistance, then you will need to consider what other help is available. You should give enough information to the person, who may have gone for help, for instance, tell him or her if the casualty is breathing or unconscious, how many casualties and what happened. Do not forget to ask the person to come back to reassure you that help is on the way. Remember to state where you are and give any landmarks that may help the emergency services.

The primary survey

If you find yourself in an emergency situation, your initial priority is to check for any dangers. Once you have established that you and your casualty are safe, your priority is the primary survey. This phase involves assessing for life threatening conditions and giving treatment as necessary.

It includes checking for any response, opening the airway, checking for breathing and observing for any bleeding (Kindleysides, 2007).

The primary survey involves a sequence of steps which can be simply remembered as **ABCDE**. This sequence of steps is a mnemonic, or a simple way for memorising essential steps in dealing with an unconscious or unresponsive patient. It is to remind you of the priorities for assessment and treatment of many acute medical situations, from basic first aid to cardiac arrest. These steps are vital for life, and each is required, in that order, for the next to be effective. It stands for **A**irway, **B**reathing and **C**irculation. However, the Resuscitation Council UK In-hospital Resuscitation guidelines (2005a) add additional steps such as **D** and **E** which are aimed primarily at healthcare professionals who are first to respond to an in-hospital cardiac arrest. It can also be applicable to other healthcare professionals in other clinical areas.

The **D** step is for **D**isability (disabilities caused by the injury, not pre-existing conditions) or **D**efibrillation (when used as a CPR protocol). Additionally, some protocols call for an **E** step to patient assessment. At this point, all protocols diverge from looking after basic life support, and are looking for underlying causes. In some protocols, there can be up to three **E**'s used. **E** can stand for **E**nvironment — only after assessing **ABCD** would you deal with environment-related symptoms or conditions such as cold and lightning. **E**xposure or **E**xamine is used mainly for ambulance level practitioners where it is important to remove clothing and other obstructions in order to assess wounds. **E**scaping air can be through a chest wound that could lead to a collapsed lung.

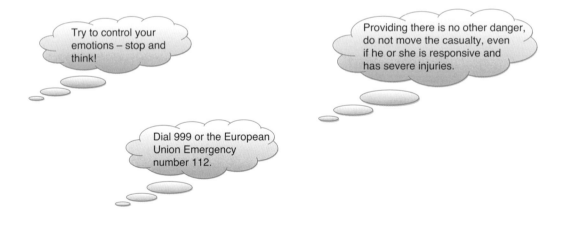

Figure 8.1 shows the student listening for any signs of breathing. Note that he is looking at the chest for any movement of the chest wall.

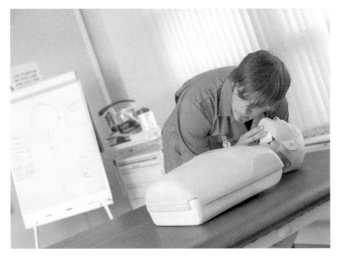

Figure 8.1   Listening for breathing

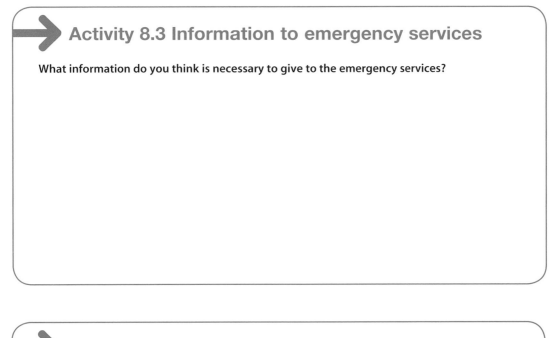

> ## Activity 8.3 Information to emergency services
>
> **What information do you think is necessary to give to the emergency services?**

> ## Activity 8.4 Do NOT do...
>
> **What do you think you should NOT do in the event of an emergency situation?**
>
> *(continued)*

> ➡️ **Activity 8.4 (*Continued*)**

If the casualty has collapsed and appears to be lifeless, an assessment following the Resuscitation Council UK guidelines (2005a) is required. This includes assessment of the airway.

- **Airway**: check that the airway is open. If the casualty is unconscious and is unresponsive, you need to make sure that the airway is clear of any obstructions, as the breaths may be faint and shallow. Obstruction of the airway can be life threatening and needs to be dealt with immediately. Place your fingers on the forehead, and using two fingers, tilt the chin up to open the airway. In this position, the weight of the tongue will force it to shift away from the back of the throat, opening the airway. Look in the mouth for any obvious obstruction and then check for normal breathing for at least 10 seconds.
  - **Look**: for any chest movement such as any accessory muscles in the neck or abdomen. Check for any discolouration of the lips — central cyanosis is a late sign of airway obstruction (Smith, 2003). An obstructed airway can occur either externally, through trauma to the face or jaw, or internally, affecting the buccal, pharynx or larynx (Dean, 2005).
  - **Listen**: for any breathing by placing your ear to their mouth and nose. Listen for any abnormal sounds such as gurgling which could indicate fluid in the upper airway, or snoring which could indicate a blockage in the upper airway in an unconscious casualty (Jevon, 2008). Normal breathing should be quiet and effortless.
  - **Feel**: can you feel the movement or air at the mouth and nose? In some environments, it may be difficult to look at the chest (particularly if it is difficult or not appropriate to expose the chest), and it may be difficult to listen if the external environment is very noisy. In such circumstances, feeling for breath and the movement of air at the nose or mouth may be the most reliable option. You can do this by placing your hand on the chest.
- **Breathing**: check for any signs of breathing. You can do this by placing your ear to the casualties' mouth looking down the body towards the chest. If you determine that the casualty is not breathing, then something may be blocking the airway. The tongue can be the most common airway obstruction in an unconscious person. Check breathing for 10 s. If the casualty is breathing normally, place in the recovery position, check for continued breathing and await assistance. Monitor their vital signs which would be their level of response by talking to them, and check their pulse and breathing regularly. If no signs of breathing, give 30 chest compressions immediately.
- **Circulation:** the UK Resuscitation Council (2005a) highlighted that there needed to be a change in the checking for circulation. This was due to evidence by Bahr *et al.* (1997) that identified that a lay person checking a carotid pulse to diagnose cardiac arrest is unreliable and time consuming, when attempted by a lay person. Subsequent studies (Hauff *et al.*, 2003) have shown that checking for breathing is also prone to error, particularly as agonal

gasps are frequently misdiagnosed as normal breathing. Agonal gasping is best described as infrequent, irregular breathing which is present in 40% of cardiac arrest casualties (Sevett, 2006). Therefore, the absence of breathing, in a non-responsive casualty, continues to be the main sign of cardiac arrest. Also highlighted is the need to identify agonal gasps as another, positive, indication to start CPR (Resuscitation Council UK guidelines, 2005a).

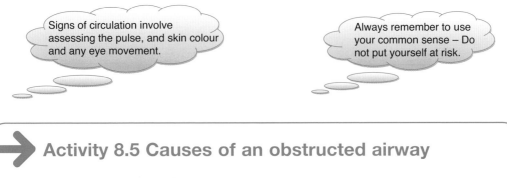

Signs of circulation involve assessing the pulse, and skin colour and any eye movement.

Always remember to use your common sense – Do not put yourself at risk.

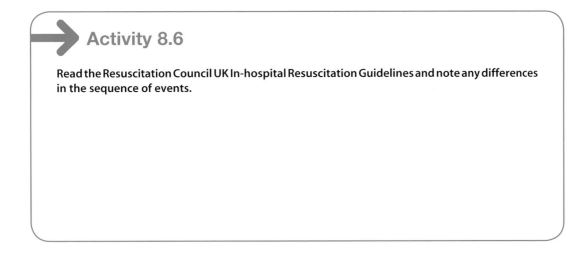

→ Activity 8.5 Causes of an obstructed airway

List some of the main causes of an obstructed airway.

In-hospital resuscitation

The Resuscitation Council UK In-hospital Resuscitation Guidelines (2005a) highlight that all healthcare professionals are trained in basic life support (BLS) techniques. These new guidelines are aimed primarily at healthcare professionals who are first to respond to an in-hospital cardiac arrest. Some of the guidelines are also applicable to healthcare professionals in other clinical settings.

→ Activity 8.6

Read the Resuscitation Council UK In-hospital Resuscitation Guidelines and note any differences in the sequence of events.

To recap, please see the summary provided in Figure 8.2.

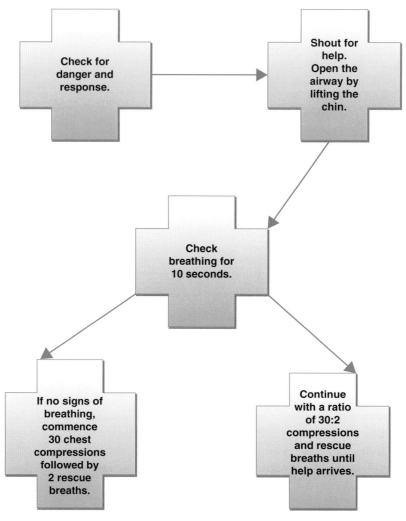

Figure 8.2   Summary of priorities in a first aid situation

The recovery position

The recovery position is a relatively simple manoeuvre to do; it is very effective and can save lives. It is vital to ensure an unconscious person is put in this position to maintain the airway. Figure 8.3 demonstrates the student maintaining the airway whilst the casualty is in the recovery position.

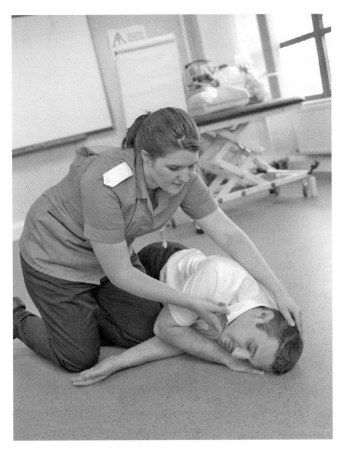

Figure 8.3   Maintaining the airway

Activity 8.7

The Resuscitation Council UK (2005a) recommend 11 steps to an effective recovery position.

Name at least five of these steps in sequential order:

1.

2.

3.

4.

5.

(Continued)

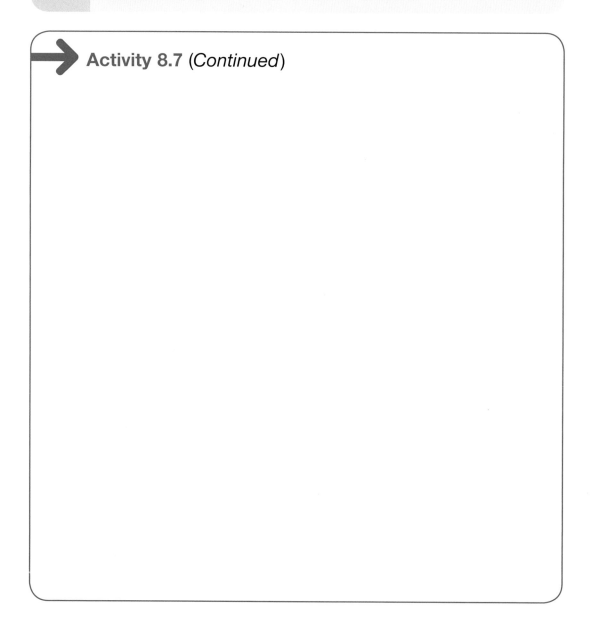

Activity 8.7 (*Continued*)

If you suspect a spinal injury, and need to put the casualty in the recovery position, get others to help you to roll using the logroll technique, keeping the spine straight, whilst steadying the head. If your casualty is not breathing normally, and your casualty is unconscious, you must commence CPR.

Cardio-pulmonary resuscitation

In order for you to have an understanding of CPR, it is important for you to understand the anatomy and physiology of the cardiac and respiratory systems. You may wish to refer to your anatomy and physiology books here.

Activity 8.8

Label the structures in the following figure.

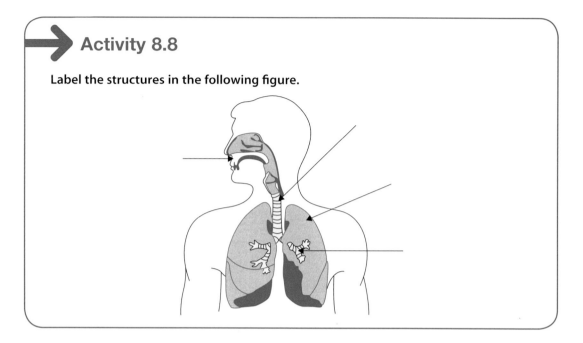

The air we breathe in travels to our lungs where oxygen is picked up by the blood and then pumped by the heart to the tissue and organs. The heart is a muscular pump that pumps blood around the body. Its primary purpose is to pump 24 hours per day, 60–80 times per minute for an adult (Sevett, 2006). The heart acts as a pump, pumping blood by muscular contractions called heartbeats to circulate the oxygen to the essential organs of the body, such as the brain, lungs, heart, kidneys and liver. When a person experiences cardiac arrest, whether due to heart failure or an injury such as near drowning, electrocution or bleeding, the heart can go from a normal beat to an arrhythmic pattern called ventricular fibrillation, and eventually ceases to beat. This prevents oxygen from circulating throughout the body, rapidly killing cells and tissue.

Essentially, **cardio-** (heart) **pulmonary** (lung) **resuscitation** is an emergency exercise that aims to restore circulation and breathing following a cardiac arrest. It is essential therefore that you ensure that the airway is open so oxygen can be inspired, thereby ensuring that gaseous exchange takes place.

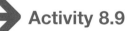 **Activity 8.9**

Listen to the audio file by St John Ambulance which will explain CPR for adults. Copy and paste the link into your URL http://www.sja.org.uk/sja/media/mp3/cpr-adult.mp3.

Starting chest compressions creates blood flow by increasing intra-thoracic pressure or directly compressing the heart (Jevon, 2008).

- Kneel by the side of the casualty.
- Place the heel of one hand in the centre of the casualty's chest.

- Place the heel of your other hand on top of the first hand.
- Interlock the fingers of your hands and ensure that pressure is not applied over the casualty's ribs.
- Do not apply any pressure over the upper abdomen or the bottom end of the bony sternum (breastbone). Place hands in the centre of the chest.
- Position yourself vertically above the casualty's chest and, with your arms straight, compress the chest 30 times pressing down on the sternum to 4–5 cm depth.
- After each compression, release all the pressure on the chest without losing contact between your hands and the sternum.
- Repeat at a rate of about 100 times a minute (a little less than two compressions a second).
- Compression and release should take an equal amount of time.

Figure 8.4 demonstrates the position of the hands in the centre of the chest in preparation for chest compressions.

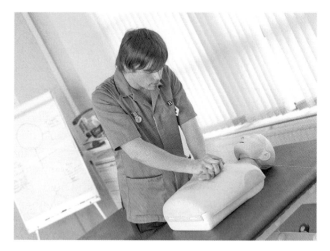

Figure 8.4   Chest compressions

Combine chest compression with rescue breaths

- After 30 compressions, open the airway again using head tilt and chin lift.
- Pinch the soft part of the casualty's nose closed, using the index finger and thumb of your hand on the forehead.
- Allow mouth to open, but maintain chin lift. Take a normal breath and place your lips around the mouth, making sure that you have a good seal.

Immediately follow the chest compressions with two rescue breaths

Blow steadily into the mouth whilst watching for the chest to rise; take about 1 second to make the chest rise as in normal breathing; this is an effective rescue breath. It is well documented that there is a reluctance to undertake mouth-to-mouth resuscitation (Resuscitation Council UK, 2005a) and this may prevent someone from attempting this process. The Resuscitation Council UK guidelines (2005a) suggest that chest-compression-only CPR may be as effective as combined ventilation and compression in the first few minutes after non-asphyxia arrest. If you feel that you are unwilling to perform rescue breaths, then you should consider doing compression-only CPR. However, combined chest compression and ventilation is the better method of CPR:

- Maintaining head tilt and chin lift, take your mouth away from the casualty and watch for the chest to fall as air comes out.
- Take another normal breath and blow into the casualty's mouth once more to give a total of two effective rescue breaths. Then return your hands without delay to the correct position on the sternum and give a further 30 chest compressions.
- Continue with chest compressions and rescue breaths in a ratio of 30:2.
- Stop to recheck the casualty only if he starts breathing **normally**; otherwise **do not interrupt resuscitation.**

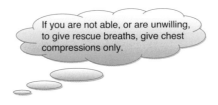

This is summarised in Figure 8.5.

Continue this cycle of 30 compressions followed by two rescue breaths.

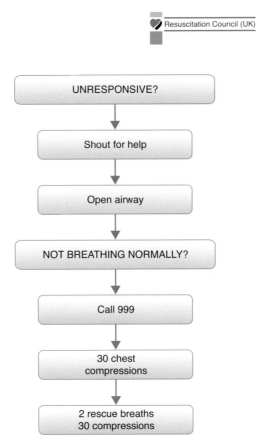

Figure 8.5   Adult basic life support

(*Source:* Reproduced with permission from the Resuscitation Council UK)

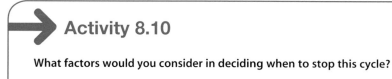

Activity 8.10

What factors would you consider in deciding when to stop this cycle?

Choking

Complete obstruction of the airway by a foreign body is a life threatening emergency and recognition is the key to a successful outcome (The Resuscitation Council UK, 2005a). Choking is usually caused by a piece of foreign matter such as food becoming lodged in a person's windpipe and is sometimes referred to as a Foreign Body Airway Obstruction (FBAO).

Activity 8.11

List here the most common signs of airway obstruction.

Because a choking casualty is fully aware that he cannot breathe normally, a sense of panic may overcome him, making assessing the situation and rescue efforts difficult. It is important to try and keep the casualty calm in order to determine whether your assistance is truly necessary or if the casualty's own coughing reflex is sufficient. However, a sudden onset of choking will cause the casualty to grasp at his neck with a panic look on his face.

It is important to ask the person if he is choking. This simple step can be deceptively effective, the casualty may be coughing violently or even gasping for air, but if he is able to answer then he is probably **not** choking. A choking casualty will not be able to speak since oxygen cannot reach his lungs, but if after asking the person if he is choking all he can do is gesture or point to his throat and you notice his face starting to turn blue, then he is most likely choking and you may need to give emergency care.

The Resuscitation Council UK guidelines (2005a) recommend the following sequence of actions:

1. If the casualty shows signs of mild airway obstruction, encourage him to continue coughing, but do nothing else.

2. If the casualty shows signs of severe airway obstruction and is conscious:

   (a) Give up to five back blows.

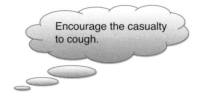

Encourage the casualty to cough.

   (b) Stand to the side and slightly behind the casualty.
   (c) Support the chest with one hand and lean the casualty well forwards, so that when the obstructing object is dislodged, it comes out of the mouth rather than goes further down the airway.
   (d) Give **up to** five sharp blows between the shoulder blades with the heel of your other hand.
   (e) Check to see if each back blow has relieved the airway obstruction.

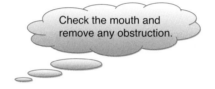

Check the mouth and remove any obstruction.

   (f) The aim is to relieve the obstruction with each blow rather than necessarily to give all five.

Figure 8.6 demonstrates the student giving back blows. Note the position of the casualty leaning forwards:

   (g) If five back blows fail to relieve the airway obstruction, give up to five abdominal thrusts (this is called the Heimlich manoeuvre).
   (h) Stand behind the casualty and put both arms round the upper part of his abdomen.
   (i) Lean the casualty forwards.
   (j) Clench your fist and place it between the umbilicus (navel) and the bottom end of the sternum (breastbone).
   (k) Grasp this hand with your other hand and pull sharply inwards and upwards.
   (l) Repeat up to five times.

3. If the obstruction is still not relieved, continue alternating five back blows with five abdominal thrusts.

4. If the casualty becomes unconscious:
   - Support the casualty carefully to the ground.

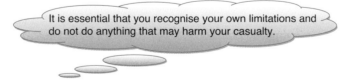

It is essential that you recognise your own limitations and do not do anything that may harm your casualty.

   - Immediately call an ambulance.
   - Begin CPR.

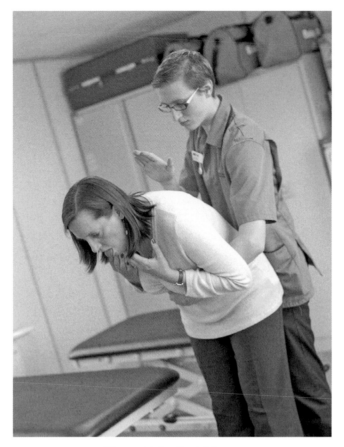

Figure 8.6   Back blows

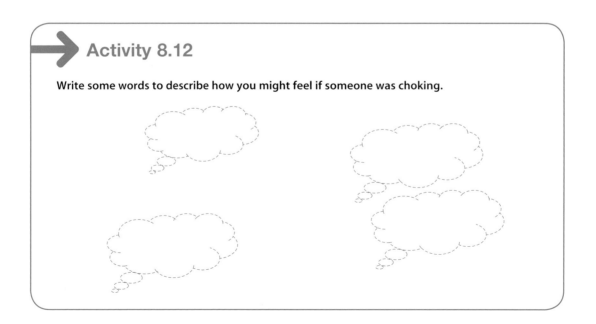

Activity 8.12

Write some words to describe how you might feel if someone was choking.

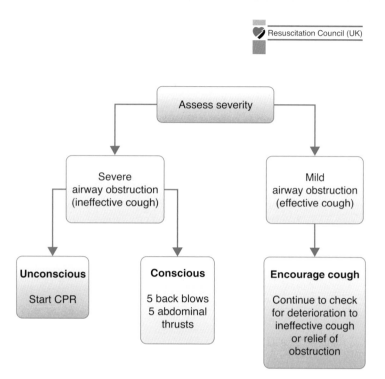

Figure 8.7   Adult choking treatment
(*Source:* Reproduced with permission from the Resuscitation Council UK)

The treatment algorithm for adult choking is based on the Resuscitation Council UK guidelines (2005a) and is summarised in Figure 8.7.

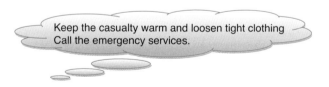

Shock

Shock is present when systemic hypoperfusion results in severe dysfunction of the vital organs (Graham and Parke, 2005) and can be defined as a state of cardiovascular dysfunction resulting in a generalised inadequacy of tissue perfusion relative to metabolic requirements (Jevon, 2008). It is a clinical syndrome and requires urgent management (Driscoll *et al.*, 2000). The main thing to remember is that your priority is to elevate the legs to get blood back to the brain. Sheppard and Wright (2003) state that the management of shock is to provide adequate perfusion to the brain and vital organs, thus ensuring an adequate transfer of gases, nutrients and waste products.

Activity 8.13 Shock

There are four classifications of shock. Write down what you think they are.

1.

2.

3.

4.

> Do not let your
> casualty eat or drink.

Activity 8.14 Signs and symptoms of shock

List the signs and symptoms of shock.

> Your aim is to improve the blood supply to the
> vital organs, such as the heart, lungs, brain,
> kidney and liver.

Treatment for shock

You should treat the underlying cause first, for instance, if the casualty is bleeding, apply pressure to the wound. Then if injuries permit, lie the casualty down and raise the legs. You can support him or her in your hands or rest him or her on a chair. Monitor and record vital signs such as pulse and respirations and remember to keep him or her talking as this is checking for levels of response. If you can feel a pulse, this will indicate that there is systolic blood pressure sufficient to achieve a basic peripheral tissue perfusion (Driscoll *et al.*, 2000). The St John Ambulance *et al.* (2006) recommend that observations should be taken at least every 10 min.

Fractures

A fracture or broken bone can be defined as a disruption of the cortex of a living bone (Jevon, 2008), but may not always be obvious as most breaks do not result in compound fractures (bone protruding through the skin). Sometimes, a fracture can be mistaken for a bruise or sprain, so it is important that you are familiar with some of the common subtypes. Those that sustain a fracture will always cause severe pain, though this pain can be confused with a sprain or dislocation as they have the same symptoms. Treatment is the same as that for a fracture (Kindleysides, 2007), which is to immobilise and send to hospital for an x-ray for a definitive diagnosis.

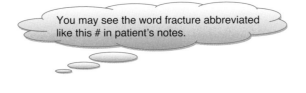

You may see the word fracture abbreviated like this # in patient's notes.

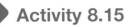

Activity 8.15

List the typical recognition features of a fracture.

Types of fractures

A fracture can be stable or unstable. This means that the bone ends do not move in a stable fracture because they are incompletely broken or jammed together (St John Ambulance *et al.*, 2006), or in an unstable fracture, the broken bones move about which can cause damage to nearby vessels, organs or tissue. There are many types of fractures which can be caused by direct or indirect force, but for the purpose of this chapter, we will discuss the two main types. These are:

- Closed fracture
- Open fracture

Activity 8.16

Listen and watch the video which describes some common fractures. Copy and paste the link into your url. http://video.about.com/orthopedics/Fractures-1.htm.

Closed fracture

This means that the bone is fractured but remains contained within the skin; therefore the bone does not penetrate the skin. However, bone ends may damage internal tissues or blood vessels, so internal bleeding may occur.

Treatment
Your priority is to

- Immobilise and support the limb to prevent further movement.
- Call the emergency services immediately at 999/112 when in Europe.
- Monitor the casualty.
- Treat for shock. Raise the legs providing this does not cause further pain.
- Calm and reassure casualty.
- Ensure that your casualty lies still.

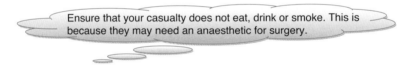

Ensure that your casualty does not eat, drink or smoke. This is because they may need an anaesthetic for surgery.

To support the limb, a bandage or splint can be applied. For lower limb fractures, a functional splint can be made of almost any material as long as it is rigid and is longer than the broken bone. To apply the splint, lay it along the broken bone and wrap it against the limb with gauze or a length of cloth, starting at a point furthest from the body. Do not wrap it too tight as this may cut off blood flow. If the break is in the upper body such as the arm, you can immobilise the arm against the body by using a sling (see Figure 8.8). A break in the lower part of the leg requires two splints, one on each side of the leg (or at least the shin). If suitable material is not available, you can use the casualty's healthy leg as a makeshift splint.

Open fracture

An open fracture (or compound fracture) is where the broken bone protrudes through the skin surface. This is an important distinction because when a broken bone penetrates the skin there is a need for immediate treatment, and an operation is often required to clean the area of the fracture. Furthermore, because of the risk of infection, there are more often problems associated with healing when a fracture is open to the skin. This type of fracture can be associated with

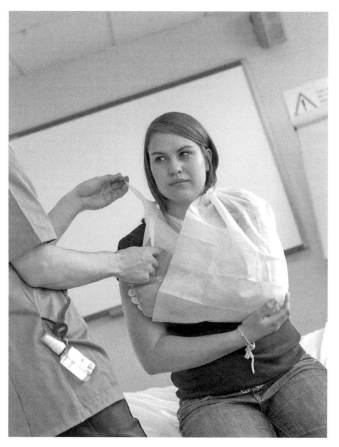

Figure 8.8   Demonstrates how a sling can immobilise the arm

haemorrhage or vascular injury (Jevon, 2008); therefore, the casualty is likely to lose blood and suffer from shock.

Treatment

- Treat the same as with closed fractures.
- Control bleeding — apply pressure if possible around the protruding bone (wear gloves if possible).
- Treat for shock.

As much as possible, keep the casualty from moving and until an ambulance arrives remember the acronym **RICE** (Jevon, 2008):

- **R** is for rest. Short-term rest eases discomfort.
- **I** is for ice — if possible apply an ice pack or ice cubes to the injured area over at least 24 h. This will keep down the swelling and reduce pain.
- **C** is for compression — if the wound is bleeding, apply pressure with a clean cloth to reduce blood flow.
- **E** is for elevation — try to keep the injured area as high above heart level as possible even when asleep (Evans and Burke, 1995). This will reduce blood flow to the injury and minimise swelling. However, do not raise the injured limb if this causes more pain.

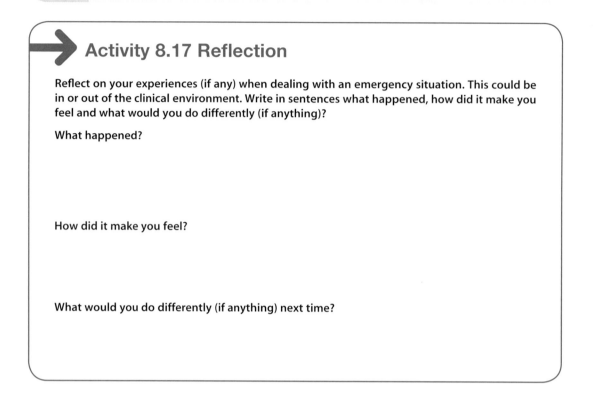

Activity 8.17 Reflection

Reflect on your experiences (if any) when dealing with an emergency situation. This could be in or out of the clinical environment. Write in sentences what happened, how did it make you feel and what would you do differently (if anything)?

What happened?

How did it make you feel?

What would you do differently (if anything) next time?

Chapter summary

Dealing with any emergency situation can be very frightening, especially if you do not know what to do, in what order and how. If you remember the basic principles of the primary survey, look for danger, that is danger to you and your casualty, and then see if there is any response by using your voice or touching the casualty. Next, you need to remember the principles of A = Airway and B = Breathing. Simply by lifting the chin and opening the airway can save a life. Ask yourself — are there any obstructions in the airway? Can you hear any breathing? What is the colour of his or her lips? Check for breathing for 10 seconds. What should you do next? Remember to remain calm when you approach the casualty and you will be able to remember all the skills that you have learnt. Send someone for help, or you go for help if others are with the casualty. There is plenty for you to do without having to commence full resuscitation. Also, remember to know your limitations.

Knowing how to give first aid treatment is a skill that needs to be learnt. It takes practice to be proficient and having confidence in your abilities helps too. Having knowledge of basic first aid skills and CPR will not only save a life but will also demonstrate competence that the public expect. Dean (2005) highlights that the public, patients and visitors have an expectation that a healthcare professional will have the competence to assist and provide first aid at the scene of any emergency. You should, however, never wear your uniform outside of the clinical area. Think about what you are telling the public if you are seen outside the clinical area in your uniform. There will be an expectation for you to assist or deliver competent first aid treatment. This of course is a pre-conceived idea that the public assume that as you are wearing a uniform you are a competent first aider. However, if you are seen to walk away from an accident when wearing a uniform, you be seen as negligent to onlookers (Kindleysides, 2007), but fear of legal recourse is no excuse for failing to provide life-saving care (Castledine, 1993).

Nurses and other healthcare professionals are not trained to be first aiders, so they would benefit from advanced first aid skills training. It is hoped that this will lead to greater skills and confidence in dealing with an emergency both in hospital and in the community.

This chapter has provided an overview of the primary survey, and the fundamental principles of first aid. The content of this chapter is by no means exhaustive as there is much more to be discussed. If this chapter has whetted your appetite to learn more, you may consider enrolling on a First Aid at Work course which is approved by the Health and Safety Executive in accordance with the Health and Safety (First Aid) Regulations 1981. This would give you a certificate and you would then be a qualified first aider. Certification is then valid for 3 years. You have attempted activities relating to the primary survey and other first aid situations. These should begin to provide you with the knowledge and skills to assist or care for casualties. You should now be able to understand these basic principles, and then apply these skills to any emergency situation in any environment. You will also begin to build on your assessment skills which will enable you to develop not only as a healthcare professional, but also as a competent and proficient person who can save a life.

Answers to Activities

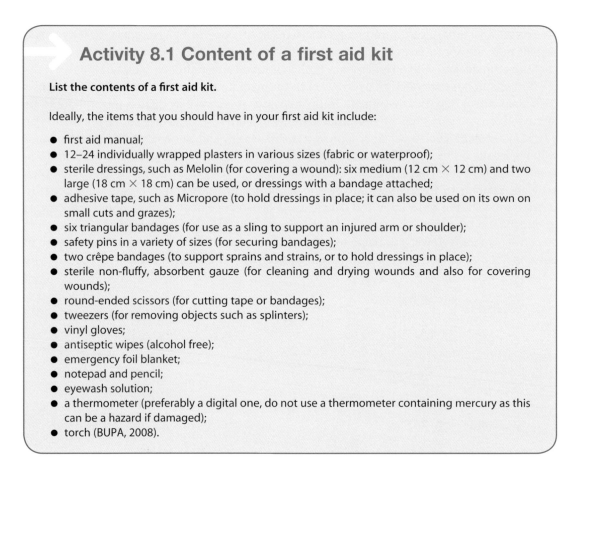

Activity 8.1 Content of a first aid kit

List the contents of a first aid kit.

Ideally, the items that you should have in your first aid kit include:

- first aid manual;
- 12–24 individually wrapped plasters in various sizes (fabric or waterproof);
- sterile dressings, such as Melolin (for covering a wound): six medium (12 cm × 12 cm) and two large (18 cm × 18 cm) can be used, or dressings with a bandage attached;
- adhesive tape, such as Micropore (to hold dressings in place; it can also be used on its own on small cuts and grazes);
- six triangular bandages (for use as a sling to support an injured arm or shoulder);
- safety pins in a variety of sizes (for securing bandages);
- two crêpe bandages (to support sprains and strains, or to hold dressings in place);
- sterile non-fluffy, absorbent gauze (for cleaning and drying wounds and also for covering wounds);
- round-ended scissors (for cutting tape or bandages);
- tweezers (for removing objects such as splinters);
- vinyl gloves;
- antiseptic wipes (alcohol free);
- emergency foil blanket;
- notepad and pencil;
- eyewash solution;
- a thermometer (preferably a digital one, do not use a thermometer containing mercury as this can be a hazard if damaged);
- torch (BUPA, 2008).

Activity 8.2 First aid containers

What do you think should be the golden rules for first aid containers?

The containers for your first aid box should be:

- clean and free from dust;
- contents protected from dust;
- made accessible if in the work place, preferably near a sink;
- green with a white cross;
- examined regularly and restocked after use (Sevett, 2006).

Activity 8.3 Information to emergency services

What information do you think is necessary to give to the emergency services?

- Your name
- The number from which you are calling
- Exact location of incident including road name and number. You can include any landmark or junction nearby.
- Time of incident
- Exact details of incident, the number of casualties, their ages if known and information about their condition.
- Details of any hazards (Jevon, 2008).

You could also consider LIONEL (Sevett, 2006):

L = Location
I = Incident
O = Other services
N = Number of casualties
E = Extent of the injuries
L = Repeat location

An example of what to say could be:

Hello, this is an emergency. I need an ambulance for 66, The Warren, Aidshire, which is near the supermarket on the corner. I have an elderly man here who is unconscious but breathing.

Activity 8.4 Do NOT do…

What do you think you should NOT do in the event of an emergency situation?

- DO NOT leave the casualty alone
- DO NOT try to make the casualty drink water
- DO NOT throw water on the casualty's face
- DO NOT prompt the casualty into a sitting position
- DO NOT try to revive the casualty by slapping the face

Activity 8.5 Causes of an obstructed airway

List some of the main causes of an obstructed airway.

- Choking — the inhalation of a foreign object such as food.
- Blockage of the larynx by the tongue
- Aspiration of gastric contents, such as blood or vomit, whilst the casualty is unconscious.
- Internal swelling of the throat, such as burns, stings, scalds or anaphylactic shock.
- Injuries to the face or jaw
- External pressure on the throat, such as hanging or strangulation (Dean, 2005).

Activity 8.6

Read the Resuscitation Council UK In-hospital Resuscitation Guidelines and note any differences in the sequence of events.

In-hospital resuscitation

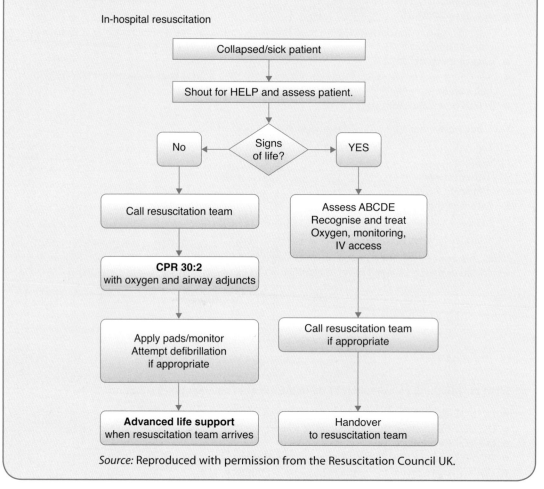

Source: Reproduced with permission from the Resuscitation Council UK.

→ **Activity 8.7**

The Resuscitation Council UK (2005) recommend 11 steps to an effective recovery position.

Name at least five of these steps in sequential order:

1. Remove the casualty's glasses.
2. Kneel besides the casualty and ensure that both the legs are straight.
3. Place casualty's arm which is nearest to you out at a right angle to the body, elbow bent with the palm facing upwards.
4. Bringing the casualty's far arm across the chest, hold the back of the hand against the casualty's cheek which is nearest to you.

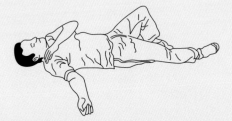

5. Using the other hand, grasp the casualty's far leg just above the knee and pull it up, keeping the foot on the ground.
6. Whilst keeping the casualty's hand pressed against the cheek, pull on the leg as a lever to roll the casualty towards you onto his or her side.
7. Adjust the casualty's upper leg, ensuring that both the hip and the knee are bent at right angles.

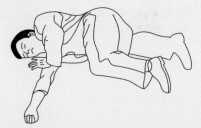

8. Tilt the casualty's head back to ensure that the airway remains patent.
9. If necessary, adjust the hand under the cheek to help ensure the head remains tilted.
10. Monitor the casualty's vital signs.
11. Monitor the peripheral circulation in the lower arm; pressure on this area should be kept to a minimum. Turn the casualty to the opposite side if the recovery position has been maintained for more than 30 min (Resuscitation Council UK, 2005a).

Activity 8.8

Label the diagram in the following figure.

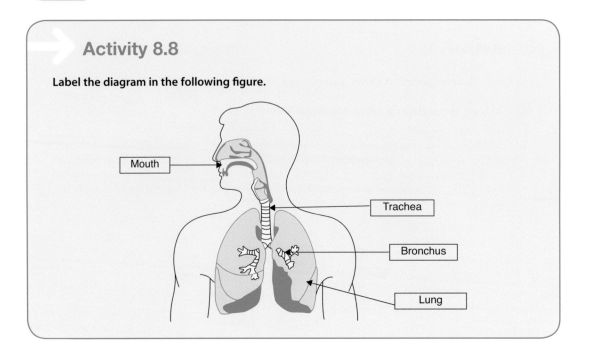

Mouth

Trachea

Bronchus

Lung

Activity 8.9

Listen to the audio file by St John Ambulance which will explain CPR for adults. Copy and paste the link into your URL http://www.sja.org.uk/sja/media/mp3/cpr-adult.mp3.

Audio file

Activity 8.10

What factors would you consider in deciding when to stop this cycle?

Factors to consider when stopping chest compressions:

- When help arrives
- When the casualty begins to breathe normally
- When you become too exhausted to continue

Activity 8.11

List here the most common signs of airway obstruction.

Signs of complete airway obstruction could be:

- Sudden inability to talk, breathe or cough.
- Maximal respiratory effort
- Development of cyanosis and clutching of the neck
- Casualty will eventually collapse and become unconscious (Jevon, 2008).

Activity 8.12

Write some words to describe how you might feel if someone was choking.

You may have used words such as 'frightened, scared, anxious, nervous, and panicky'.

Activity 8.13 Shock

There are four classifications of shock. Write down what you think they are.

Four classifications of shock are:

1. **Hypovolaemic shock:** loss of circulating blood or volume caused by haemorrhage, burns, severe vomiting and diarrhoea and intestinal obstruction.
2. **Cardiogenic shock:** cardiac pump failure, causes include myocardial infarction, cardiac arrhythmias and myocarditis.
3. **Distributive shock:** abnormality of the peripheral circulation, causes include sepsis and anaphylaxis.
4. **Obstructive shock:** mechanical obstruction to cardiac output, causes include pulmonary embolism and cardiac tamponade (Hinds and Watson, 1999).

Activity 8.14 Signs and symptoms of shock

List the signs and symptoms of shock.

- Tachycardia (fast heart beat)
- Cold and clammy skin
- Pallor-pale to look at
- Tachypnoea (fast respiratory rate)
- Yawning and sighing
- Restlessness and agitation (British Red Cross, 2003)

Other symptoms may include nausea and thirst, rapid shallow breathing and eventually leading to unconsciousness as the oxygen supply diminishes.

Activity 8.15

List the typical recognition features of a fracture.
Typical recognition features of a fracture are:

- Immediate and excessive swelling
- Injured area appears deformed
- The extremities of the injured limb may turn blue or are numb to the touch
- Excessive pain caused by even the slightest movement
- Potential signs of shock, especially if the fracture is to the thigh bone or pelvis (St John Ambulance et al., 2006).

Activity 8.16

Listen and watch the video which describes some common fractures. Copy and paste the link into your url. http://video.about.com/orthopedics/Fractures-1.htm.

This activity is for you to listen/watch the video.

Activity 8.17 Reflection

Reflect on your experiences (if any) when dealing with an emergency situation. This could be in or out of the clinical environment. Write in sentences what happened, how did it make you feel and what would you do differently (if anything)?

This is your personal experience of caring for a casualty in an emergency situation. Reflect your own personal feelings in relation to your learning needs. You may have more than one learning need; hence you could use the same subheadings to address the issues.

Activity 8.17 (*Continued*)

What happened?

● Describe the scenario briefly relating to your learning need.

How did it make you feel?

● What was good or bad about it?
● Did you have adequate underpinning knowledge to carry out the care?
● If you had previous experience of similar situation, was it useful this time?

What would you do differently (if anything) next time?

● Has this personal experience prepared you to do further reading?

This is only a guide towards your own reflection. Please use the subheadings to meet your own learning needs.

References

Bahr, J., Klingler, H., Panzer, W., Rode, H. and Kettler, D. (1997) Skills of lay people in checking the carotid pulse. *Resuscitation* **35**, 23–26.

BBC News Online (1999) Nurses' first aid skills declining. June 18. http://news.bbc.co.uk/1/hi/health/372439.stm (accessed 26 June 2008).

British Red Cross (2003) *Practical First Aid* (Middlesex: Dorling Kindersley).

BUPA (2008) http://hcd2.bupa.co.uk/fact_sheets/html/first_aid.html#1 (accessed 26 June 2008).

Castledine, G. (1993) Ethical implications of first aid. *British Journal of Nursing* **2** (4), 239–241.

Dean, R. (2005) Emergency first aid for nurses. *Nursing Standard* **20** (6), 57–65.

Dimond, B. (2005) Dilemma. *Nursing Times* **101** (23), 42.

Dimond, B. (2008) *Legal Aspects of Nursing*, 5th edn (Harlow: Pearson Education).

Driscoll, P., Skinner, D. and Earlem, R. (2000) *ABC of Major Trauma*, 3rd edn (London: BMJ Publishing Group).

Evans, R. and Burke, D. (1995) *Key Topics in Accident and Emergency Medicine* (Oxford: BIOS).

Ford, P., McCormack, B., Wills, T. and Dewing, J. (2000) Defining the boundaries: nursing and personal care. *Nursing Standard* **15** (3), 43–45.

Graham, C.A. and Parke, T.R.J. (2005) Critical care in the emergency department: shock and circulatory support. *Emergency Medicine Journal* **22** (1), 17–21.

Hauff, S.R., Rea, T.D., Culley, L.L., Kerry, F., Becker, L. and Eisenberg, M.S. (2003) Factors impeding dispatcher-assisted telephone cardiopulmonary resuscitation. *Annual Emergency Medical* **42**, 731–737.

Hinds, C.J. and Watson, D. (1999) ABC of intensive care: circulatory support. *British Medical Journal* **318**, 1749-1752.

Jevon, P. (2008) *Emergency Care: First Aid for Nurses — A Practical Guide* (London: Churchill Livingstone).

Kindleysides, D. (2007) First aid: basic procedures for nurses. *Nursing Standard* **21** (18), 48–57.

McBean, S. (2002) First aid training: developing the debate. *Nursing in Practice* **6**, 39–41.

Nursing and Midwifery Council (2004) *The NMC Code of Professional Conduct: Standards for Conduct, Performance and Ethics* (London: Nursing and Midwifery Council).

Nursing and Midwifery Council (2008) *The Code: Standards of Conduct, Performance and Ethics for Nurses and Midwives* (London: Nursing and Midwifery Council).

Resuscitation Council UK (2005a) Resuscitation guidelines: adult basic life support. www.resus.org.uk (accessed 10 July 2008).

Resuscitation Council UK (2005b) Resuscitation guidelines: in-hospital resuscitation. www.resus.org.uk (accessed 10 July 2008).

Resuscitation Council UK (2008) Cardiopulmonary resuscitation: standards for clinical practice and training. www.resus.org.uk (accessed 10 July 2008).

Sevett, S. (2006) *First Aid at Work. A Text for All HSE Approved and Recognised Courses and a Reference in Particular, for Qualified First Aiders*, 4th edn (Doncaster: Highfield.co.uk Ltd).

Sheppard, M. and Wright, M. (2003) *Principles and Practice of High Dependency Nursing* (London: Balliere Tindall).

Smith, G. (2003) *ALERT: Acute Life Threatening Events Recognition and Treatment* (Portsmouth: University of Portsmouth).

St John Ambulance, St Andrew's Ambulance Association and British Red Cross (2006) *First Aid Manual*, 8th revised edn (London: Dorling Kindersley).

Wardrope, J. and Mackenzie, R. (2004) The ABC of community emergency care: 2. The system of assessment and care of the primary survey positive patient. *Emergency Medicine Journal* **21** (2), 216–225.

Further reading

Health and Safety Executive (2008) http://www.hse.gov.uk/ (accessed 10 July 2008).

Test your knowledge by attempting the first aid quiz on the following BBC website. Click on 'Test your skills' on the left-hand side of the screen: http://www.bbc.co.uk/health/first_aid/skills_test/index.shtml or try this one http://www.firstaidquiz.com/cgi-bin/quiz/index.pl

Useful websites

St John Ambulance: http://www.sja.org.uk/sja/

The Red Cross: http://www.redcrossfirstaidtraining.co.uk/

The Health and Safety Executive: http://www.hse.gov.uk/

The First Aid Cafe: http://www.firstaidcafe.co.uk/

BBC Health/First Aid: http://www.bbc.co.uk/health/first_aid/index.shtml

The UK Resuscitation Council: http://www.resus.org.uk/siteIndx.htm

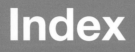

Index

Notes: *t* and *f* at the end of page numbers refer to tables and figures respectively.